LIZ EARLE

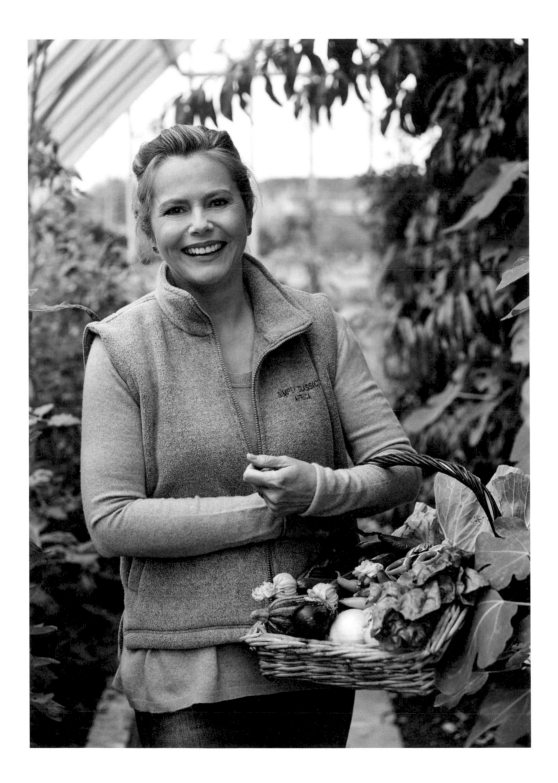

LIZ EARLE

THE ULTIMATE GUIDE TO LOOKING AND FEELING
YOUR RADIANT BEST THROUGHOUT THE
PERIMENOPAUSE, MENOPAUSE AND BEYOND

First published in Great Britain in 2018 by Orion Spring
an imprint of The Orion Publishing Group Ltd
Carmelite House, 50 Victoria Embankment
London EC4Y 0DZ

An Hachette UK Company

5 7 9 10 8 6 4

Photographer: Dan Jones
Creative Director: Helen Ewing
Designer: Clare Sivell
Project Editor: Olivia Morris
Home Economist and Food Stylist: Natalie Thomson
Props Stylist: Tamzin Ferdinando
Nutritional analysis calculated by: Fiona Hunter BSc (hons) Nutrition, Diploma Dietetics

Every effort has been made to ensure that the information in the book is accurate.
The information in this book may not be applicable in each individual case so it is advised
that professional medical advice is obtained for specific health matters and before changing
any medication or dosage. Neither the publisher nor author accepts any legal responsibility
for any personal injury or other damage or loss arising from the use of the information in
this book. In addition, if you are concerned about your diet or exercise regime and wish to
change them, you should consult a health practitioner first.

A CIP catalogue record for this book is available from the British Library.

ISBN: 978 1 4091 6418 0

Contents

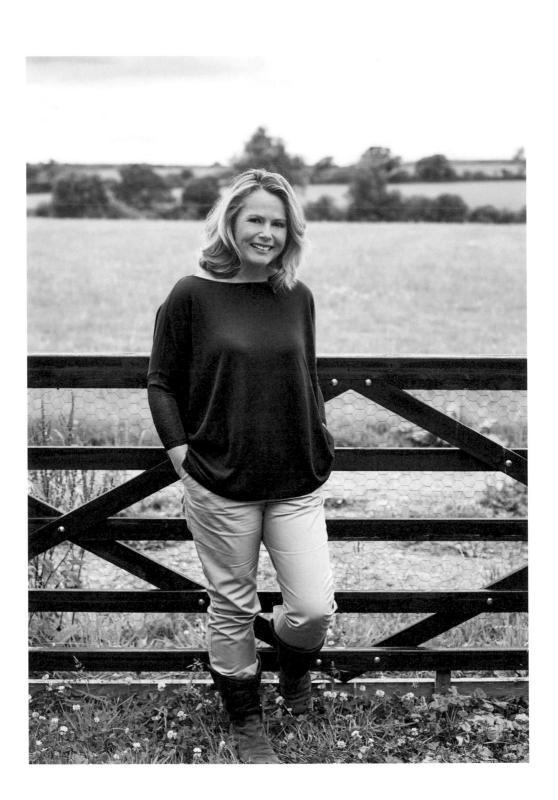

Introduction

Over the last thirty years of writing about health and wellbeing, I've championed subjects that have been largely overlooked – such as gut health in my most recent book, *The Good Gut Guide* – but nothing prepared me for what I was to discover when I started to research and write about the menopause.

Like most women, I had no real concept of what the menopause would be like until I started to consider my own personal journey, and I found it baffling that there was so little information available to me and the millions of others who were at a similar stage of life. Advice was muddled, contradictory and very often failed to explain what was happening in the body, not to mention why, and the solutions offered were too simplistic and involved far too many 'do nots' when I was seeking positive, practical information.

I couldn't believe how rarely the menopause is talked about in the media (unless, of course, it's to poke fun – cue tired-looking woman fanning herself, sweating). Discussion of it should actually start as a subject in fertility clinics or antenatal classes – but of course it doesn't – so women can find themselves with a young family, hurtling straight into the perimenopause or menopause. Here comes one of the many myths to be debunked: having a baby postpones the menopause. It does not.

When I spoke to friends about the menopause I found that many of them, left to believe the many myths and untruths, were confused by the details of this complex, but completely natural process. Why is there such a shocking lack of support? We talk so openly about pregnancy and childbirth, but when it comes to an equally important phase in every woman's life post forty there is an audible silence.

Most of us who enter the menopause at average age find ourselves in the sandwich generation – running busy lives, raising teenage children and looking out for elderly parents while also working. We may not realise that juggling so much puts us under enormous pressure. Female friends in their forties are amazed and surprised when I say that their sleeplessness, tiredness and low mood are most likely caused by shifting hormones. And, in the great majority of cases, these symptoms can be very easily treated, effectively and safely.

With little clear guidance about what to expect during 'the change' (an ominous phrase popularised by an older generation), it's easy to see why many women feel isolated and in many cases bewildered, miserable and, worst of all, embarrassed by how they feel. Besides the physical symptoms, the emotional and psychological aspects of this time of life can leave even the most capable feeling vulnerable and useless. Many women don't realise the adverse effect the menopause can have on their lives at home and at work.

Examples of this include a loss of confidence and feeling tearful at the slightest upset. Equally sudden is weight gain (usually a good 7lb) around the tummy that will not budge! Middle-age spread is a real thing. Anxiety is often a consequence and you may start waking at 4 a.m., heart racing, body on fire, and be unable to sleep. These are just a few of the tell-tale signs of the menopause, which can begin in your mid-forties while you're still having periods and not even thinking about 'the change'. Encouragingly, around one in five women do not have any symptoms at all. However, most of us do and around one in four will have symptoms so severe they affect their quality of life. The official 'menopause' is classified by doctors as coming after a full twelve months without a period. The time leading up to this is called the 'perimenopause', which can last from two months to ten years, and is the crucial time to be reading this book.

I hope this book will also be invaluable for the 3.5 million or so fifty-plus women who are in employment in the UK and are sadly neglected in this area of their health. If we do the maths, we know the menopause affects more working women than it has ever done in the past, because we are all working longer, retiring later and most of us don't anticipate how long symptoms of the menopause might last. It's perfectly normal to experience hot flushes for more than ten years (so all the more reason to give HRT a try!).

As recently as two generations ago, the menopause was a milestone in women's lives associated with being over the hill and middle-aged. Such negative connotations were reinforced by the stigma attached to it, which somehow made it shameful or embarrassing to talk about. It's worth remembering at this point that at the beginning of the twentieth century, life expectancy for women was fifty-five, meaning that they either didn't reach the menopause or had a very short experience of it.

Nowadays the vast majority of us will live for thirty to forty years after the menopause. So, my advice is to see this time of life as a good moment to take stock and begin to appreciate who we have become and what we may still achieve and do – or even change. Thankfully, as more and more successful, high-profile women reach the age of menopause and talk about its impact, it must surely become less of a taboo subject.

For not only can the menopause have a profound – and in all senses life-changing – effect on us, it also has an impact on our relationships with spouses, partners, children, family, friends and colleagues. And if they, too, can gain insight into what exactly is going on with us during the menopause, then they will be much better placed to offer support.

I'd like to encourage us all to talk openly about the challenges (and there are quite a few) and share solutions. My aim with this book is to explore an area I personally find fascinating – I'm in my mid-fifties – and to impart the knowledge I've built up over decades of talking and listening to health and wellbeing professionals. I'd like to offer, both to those who may be years away from the menopause and to those in the eye of the storm, a wealth of healthy advice backed up by the most up-to-date, trusted research. I'd like everyone to feel supported, so no matter what the menopause may bring at least they feel armed with wise and accurate information.

Of course, I don't want to sound overly pessimistic. It's perfectly possible to breeze through the menopause even when others are completely floored by it – as with pregnancy and childbirth, no two experiences are the same. In fact, I'd like to make the menopause something as widely talked about as childbirth – and even celebrated. Why has the menopause become steeped in so much negativity? I hope everyone who reads this book will feel confident they have the tools to feel and look their radiant best. And more than that, I want our daughters to embrace the menopause as simply another phase in their lives that is both natural and liberating.

You'll find guidance here on how to balance hormones, the importance of a nourishing diet, the myths and facts about HRT, osteoporosis and how to optimise bone health. As you might expect, I'll also show you how to take special care of your skin and hair, what to do about weight gain and how to boost overall energy, emotional wellbeing and self-esteem.

As part of this, I've also created sixty delicious menopause-friendly recipes to introduce into your diet which can be enjoyed year-round by all the family. I've provided useful nutritional advice along the way and included calorie counts per serving (where ranges are given, the smaller number of calories relates to the larger number of servings) as well as these symbols for:

V VEGETARIAN

DF DAIRY-FREE

GF GLUTEN-FREE

I am so grateful to the many leading experts in this field who gave so much of their valuable time to share their experience and wisdom so freely. I am especially thankful to all those mentioned in the health professional credits on page 232.

I hope you find your new-found knowledge a genuine help, and take away some inspiration, words of comfort and encouragement, to make this phase of your life as happy, healthy and enjoyable as it can possibly be. I'd love to hear how you get on, so do please share your stories and experiences along the way, joining in the conversation on social media using the hashtag #goodmenopause, to encourage and inspire others through a better menopause journey – you'll find all my contact details on page 240.

With love,

Liz x

Liz Earle MBE
Lizearlewellbeing.com

PART ONE:
THE GUIDE

CHAPTER ONE:
Perimenopause 40+

Never heard the term 'perimenopause'? Well, read on … If you're a 40+ female, it's quite possibly happening to you right now. According to the World Health Organization, out of a global population of 3.5 billion there'll be 1.1 billion women aged fifty or over by 2025, *all* of whom will have already experienced the perimenopause.

Let's start with the definitions. The 'menopause', often described as a phase, is actually the name given to the year after a woman's last ever period. After this date we are 'postmenopausal'.

The perimenopause technically means the time of transition to the menopause, and it's as individual as a thumbprint. It may last a few months or even up to ten years and all of these time spans are considered completely normal in medical terms. There is no right or wrong – and, annoyingly, still no definitive test to predict precisely at what point we may be on our journey or how long it might go on for.

The average length of the perimenopause is around four years. Hormonal changes can fluctuate so dramatically in our forties that PMS symptoms such as anxiety and water retention can easily be mistaken for the perimenopause and vice versa. One fact to be aware of is that the more rapidly the ovaries fail, the greater the likelihood of severe symptoms. For example, if you find your PMS symptoms last all month then they're more likely to actually be symptoms of the perimenopause.

I find it frustrating that so little is talked about this time – as many unpleasant mid-life female ailments are actually caused by the perimenopause (which many women might not be aware of). These include tiredness, irritability, anxiety, sleepless nights, bladder problems, low libido, sagging skin and weight gain. Sounds familiar? You're not alone and, fortunately, there's plenty that can be done to help.

Despite puberty starting earlier nowadays, this has curiously made no difference to the age at which the menopause begins (average age fifty-one), with symptoms usually starting from around the age of forty-five onwards. However, women of forty and over now have a higher fertility rate than women under twenty – a figure last recorded in the 1940s – and the number of babies being born to women over forty has risen by more than a third.[1] Of course, this wonderful news means we're healthy and fertile for longer, so can reproduce later in life, but as a result we're more likely to be juggling younger childcare needs with our own perimenopausal symptoms.

Premature ovarian insufficiency

If the menopause is experienced before the age of forty, it's known as premature ovarian failure (POF), or primary ovarian insufficiency (POI), a condition characterised by the loss of functioning ovaries. There are two main complications relating to POI – one is related to infertility and the second to a greater risk of developing the serious and potentially life-threatening health conditions seen in some postmenopausal women, such as heart disease, osteoporosis and dementia.

In POI, the ovaries do not completely fail but their function can fluctuate over time, occasionally resulting in a period, ovulation or even pregnancy, sometimes several years after diagnosis.

Some women with POI are able to conceive – between 5 and 10 per cent. Although most women with POI experience symptoms of the menopause, around one in four have no symptoms other than having irregular or no periods.

The most common way of diagnosing POI is by having a blood test, so do see your GP if this is a concern. If you are diagnosed with POI, it is important hormone treatment is offered (HRT or the contraceptive pill) up to the natural age of menopause (fifty-one) to replace the hormones that the body would otherwise be producing. Without hormonal treatment, there is a greater risk of developing conditions such as osteoporosis and cardiovascular disease (CVD), so early intervention is key. It's also important to stress there are *no risks* attached to taking HRT when young.

Early menopause

If the menopause occurs before the age of forty-five, it's medically classed as early menopause and affects around 10 per cent of women.

It's unclear what triggers early menopause but studies so far conclude that women who've never had children, or who smoke, live at high altitude, have or have had eating disorders, sudden trauma or a history of depression are at greater risk. There is also a genetic link, so it is worth discussing with female relatives to assess the level of risk.

Certain conditions and medical procedures can also bring about an early menopause, such as the removal of the ovaries, radiotherapy or chemotherapy treatment. A hysterectomy removes the entire uterus and may trigger early menopause, even if the ovaries are left intact. This is because although the ovaries will still produce oestrogen, the amount will be much smaller, prompting an earlier than average menopause.

Early menopause leads to a 50 per cent higher risk of coronary heart disease and nearly a 25 per cent higher risk of cardiovascular death than for those whose menopause occurs later, according to a review of thirty-two studies from Erasmus University Medical Centre in Rotterdam, reported in *JAMA Cardiology*, involving more than 310,000 women. The findings highlighted the cardiovascular risk factors around the perimenopause and menopausal transition, and suggested the need for CVD risk assessment in those women.

One bit of good news was that no link was found between early-onset menopause and an increased risk of stroke. As such, scientists are unable to say definitively whether our reproductive system influences our cardiovascular health or cardiovascular disease is influencing the ovaries.

Of course, identifying our last ever period is only easy in hindsight, given how erratic cycles can become during the perimenopause leading up to this point. Periods may vanish for six months at a time only to return unexpectedly, as if they've never been away, or cycles may become longer or shorter, while bleeding may become heavier or lighter. You may find that symptoms such as hot flushes, palpitations or anxiety start suddenly alongside your periods, only to disappear, leaving you feeling bewildered and wondering, *is this the end*?

To prevent any late life surprises (my last child was born just a few weeks shy of my forty-eighth birthday), doctors recommend using contraception for at least a year after what we believe is our final period if over the age of fifty and for two years if under the age of fifty. And it's worth keeping tampons or similar in your handbag too, as cycle dates can shift.

It may feel as though men have comparatively little to worry about at this age, but research shows that male fertility also plummets after forty – those who wait until then to start a family run a higher risk of their partner having a miscarriage because the quality of their sperm is lower.

Puberty and menopause link

This should be of interest to all mothers with teenage daughters – the largest study of its kind (50,000 postmenopausal women)[2] across the world found that there was a link between girls starting their periods early (before age twelve) and them having their last period before turning forty-five. The knock-on effect of this is more women having premature menopause and an increase in fertility problems as a result.

Among the study group, the average age of first periods was thirteen and the last period was about fifty. However, 14 per cent of girls, on average, had their first period before they were twelve, and 10 per cent had their last period before they turned forty-five. A deep delve into the figures by Gita Mishra at the University of Queensland, Australia, revealed that those early starters were 31 per cent more likely to have an early menopause, between the ages of forty and forty-four.

Of the women who had their first period when they were thirteen, only 1.8 per cent had premature menopause (before the age of forty), and 7.2 per cent reached menopause early. But in women who had their first period when they were eleven or younger, 3.1 per cent had premature menopause, and 8.8 per cent went through it early.

Why early starters may need early families

The study also concluded that women without children who had their first period before age twelve were five times more likely to reach menopause prematurely than those with two or more children, who started their periods aged twelve or more.

The women reported difficulty falling pregnant, which suggests a link between early menstruation, infertility and premature menopause. If a woman goes through the menopause in her thirties, this means her fertility could start to drop off in her twenties – it sounds dramatic but this could have a major influence on the life plans of future generations in terms of when they decide to have a family.[3]

Global differences

Not only do we each have a unique experience of the menopause, there are global differences in the onset of perimenopause, too. A survey of more than 4,000 Japanese women aged forty-five to fifty-five confirmed the link between diet and the timing of the menopause. High calcium and soya intakes were significantly associated with the menopause happening at a later age, while the opposite was true of those with higher intakes of fat, cholesterol and coffee.[4]

Our hormone history

The complexity and extreme sensitivity of our hormonal system can easily be disrupted by the slightest physical or emotional disturbance, which is why balancing our hormones in the perimenopause is essential. It's worth having a quick refresher on how the whole cycle works to understand the subtle changes the perimenopause brings – so here's the biology bit:

Women are born on average with a million oocytes or eggs and that supply begins to fall away drastically around the age of thirty-five, so by the time we're in our forties, the numbers may be as low as a thousand and then none at all after the menopause. The menstrual cycle begins with the pituitary gland releasing female hormones (follicular stimulating hormone FSH and leuteinising hormone LH) into the bloodstream each month, which triggers our ovaries to produce oestrogen and progesterone.

Oestrogen

Oestrogen is not a single hormone – there are three main types – but scientists have actually identified at least six.

- Oestradiol (E2) is the dominant oestrogen produced by the ovaries.

- Oestrone (E1) occurs when the liver converts oestradiol to oestrone and is present post-menopause.

- Oestriol (E3) is the weakest source of oestrogen until pregnancy, when the placenta produces vast quantities to protect the foetus.

Each ovary contains follicles where the eggs grow, thanks to the follicle stimulating hormone (FSH) which triggers the release of oestrogen inside the developing follicle, while a second hormone, luteinising hormone (LH), encourages further growth of the follicle and stimulates ovulation mid-cycle.

During ovulation, the follicle bursts and releases the mature egg into the fallopian tubes, while the empty follicle develops into a mass of tissue called the *corpus luteum*, which releases progesterone and oestrogen.

After ovulation, the *corpus luteum* produces progesterone, which causes the womb lining to thicken in preparation for a fertilised egg to implant. During this luteal phase, if the egg is fertilised by sperm and embeds in the womb, the *corpus luteum* continues to produce progesterone to keep the pregnancy on track until the placenta develops enough to take over the production of progesterone for the rest of the pregnancy.

I like to think of oestrogen as also being the beauty hormone – everything about being feminine and female comes largely down to this hormone. It keeps our hair glossy, eyes bright at ovulation (some say they can detect early pregnancy by seeing it in the eyes), it plumps skin, boosts libido and is responsible for the maintenance of our whole reproductive system.

Imagine, then, how things might change as the hormone-stimulating signals from our ovaries to the brain start to fail during the perimenopause until progesterone is no longer produced (as a result of a lack of oestrogen). It's no wonder we start to notice tiny, almost imperceptible differences in how we feel – and look – before the main symptoms kick in.

The bladder, blood vessels, bones, brain, breasts, skin, heart, liver, urinary tract, hair, mucous membranes and pelvic muscles all contain oestrogen receptors. This means that they all need oestrogen for regular cell function – when levels plummet, we're likely to experience symptoms throughout our entire body! (See next chapter.)

Beyond hormones

Given that (with luck) we're likely to be alive for a long time post menopause – about a third of our lives – the best approach is to plan well in advance by appreciating exactly how our body is changing, how to balance our hormones and how to optimise our chances of having a healthy, happy, menopause. Like most busy working mothers, I'm the first to find myself at the bottom of my own to-do list (if on it at all, frankly) but the perimenopause is a good time to take a deep breath and examine your life so far. If you can prioritise your own health and wellbeing then in doing so you may help prevent chronic or serious illness further down the line.

Be prepared

With current government messages urging us all to take more responsibility for our own health and self-care, it's really useful if you now start keeping notes on your blood pressure and body mass index (BMI), then update them at least annually, so any variations can be monitored by your GP.

Are there any hereditary diseases running through the family and, if so, at what age did they begin? For example, is there any history of osteoporosis or CVD? It's important to understand any risk factors, because although women's chances of having a heart attack before the menopause are much lower than a man's they suddenly become much higher after the menopause.

An estimated 40 per cent of cancers could be prevented with lifestyle changes and it's during our forties and fifties that positive steps can be taken to lower the risk of cancer and chronic diseases, such as type 2 diabetes, CVD, osteoporosis and dementia.

KEEP ACTIVE It's not only our genes that play a huge role in how we age but our lifestyles too, as a 2013 University College London study found when they monitored the exercise habits of those in their sixties and concluded that those who exercised achieved healthy ageing and were seven times more likely to prevent serious illness than those who didn't.[5]

WEIGHT MANAGEMENT should be at the top of the agenda, as one in twenty cases of cancer is linked to being overweight or obese, and being overweight can cause thirteen types of cancer according to Cancer Research UK. Anyone who notices they are becoming apple-shaped (otherwise known as middle-age spread) really does need to tackle this now as increased belly fat is specifically linked to bowel, kidney, pancreatic and breast cancers. Scientists are unsure why, but it may be to do with how quickly certain chemicals from fat enter the bloodstream.

ORAL HEALTH also needs to be a priority now as the gums and tissue in our mouths start to show signs of receding. As we get older we produce less saliva, this allows bacteria to stick to our teeth and gums, making them more vulnerable to decay. Studies reveal a link between dental plaque and the plaque that forms in the arteries resulting in atherosclerosis, a major factor in CVD. It may sound strange, but if there's a history of CVD in the family, it's advisable to see a dental hygienist every six months (or even three months) in order to keep plaque under control.

EYE CHECKS will detect any changes in vision such as presbyopia (otherwise known as 'old sight'), which results in the need for reading glasses and usually coincides with the perimenopause. It's a good time to talk to your optician if you wear contact lenses as you may experience reduced tolerance to them due to 'dry eye syndrome' during the perimenopause, which can cause eye irritation and itchiness. You may need to start wearing your glasses more and limit use of contact lenses. Why? Falling hormones affect the ocular tissues and the production of tears. You may also notice symptoms such as blurred vision, burning eyes and a sense of having something in the eye.

Here are a few tips:

- Keep a bottle of lubricating eye drops in your bag – especially if staring at a computer for any length of time.

- Invest in a pair of good-quality sunglasses to help protect against cataracts and age-related macular degeneration.

- Make it a habit to wear sunglasses on bright and windy days to avoid eyes feeling dry and sensitive.

- Those who drink kefir regularly (a probiotic super-yoghurt) often report improvements in eye health.

HEARING LOSS should be monitored by an audiologist – especially as research shows that 40 per cent of those over fifty have some kind of hearing loss (and 70 per cent by the age of seventy). Oestrogen has a protective effect on the auditory system and a study in Sweden revealed that the menopause acts a trigger for relatively rapid age-related hearing decline in healthy women, starting in the left ear.[6]

If there's a history of congenital hearing loss, this may start to take effect from your mid-forties onwards. Yet another lesser-known symptom of declining levels of oestrogen in the body.

Protect hearing as much as possible by avoiding noisy environments and wearing ear protection on planes, when using a lawn mower and at musical concerts. Play It Down is a free iPhone and iPad app which allows users to assess their hearing ability and noisy environments.

GUT HEALTH Increasing scientific and medical research is proving that gut health has the greatest and most significant influence on mood, emotions and overall mental wellbeing. Depression used to be linked to low levels of serotonin in the brain (the neurotransmitter often credited with making us happy), but it's now known that up to 90 per cent of this mood-regulating chemical is actually produced in the gut. Keeping our levels of beneficial bacteria high is now even more important than ever (you may be interested in my earlier book, *The Good Gut Guide*, where I explore this fascinating subject in great detail).

Unfortunately, our levels of friendly bacteria in the gut can drop after the age of fifty-five, especially in the large intestine. As a result, we're more likely to suffer from poor digestion, food intolerances and a generally increased risk of gut disease. Constipation is more likely as we age, as the flow of digestive juices from the stomach, liver, pancreas and small intestine slows down, making it more important than ever to keep well hydrated and to eat unprocessed, fresh fruits and vegetables and plenty of fibre. I'm a big fan of taking multi-strain probiotic supplements (at any age) and a daily helping of plain live yoghurt and kefir, is top of my menopausal foodie checklist too (see page 218 for my kefir recipe).

LOVE YOUR LIVER It may be the largest single organ in the body but few of us recognise it as the central organ of metabolism. When we relax or sleep, a quarter of the body's blood is stored there. Our hard-working liver receives fresh arterial blood and blood-carrying products of digestion from the intestine and also identifies toxic substances (such as alcohol), which it converts into harmless waste, thus gaining a reputation as the body's waste disposal unit.

Given that the liver has the task of processing excess hormones, I like to give it a much-needed boost by including cleansing juices and foods such as artichokes, asparagus, beetroots, carrots and garlic into many everyday dishes and recipes. One herb that also works wonders in supporting the liver is milk thistle, which encourages detoxification, plus it's an excellent hangover helper … You'll find it in good health food shops or online, available as a dried herb, herbal tincture or in capsule form.

STOP SMOKING I don't need to remind anyone about the extremely detrimental effects smoking has on our health – not just on lungs, skin, oral health and eyes, but also on fertility. Numerous studies link infertility to smoking, as chemicals in nicotine reduce ovarian function.[7]

According to the Mayo Clinic, women who smoke regularly may also start the menopause a year or two earlier than women who do not. It also found that those who continue to smoke post-menopause are at an increased risk of breast cancer compared to non-smokers – and their skin ages faster. All in all, it is truly best to stub it out.

What to drink

My girlfriends and I used to enjoy more than just the occasional glass of wine, but our tolerance to alcohol has definitely gone down. Why? During the perimenopause and beyond, the body's water content is reduced, so any alcohol consumed is more concentrated in the blood and therefore more potent. Swiftly matching each glass of alcohol drunk with a glass of water is an excellent way to help avoid this.

I can't emphasise enough just how much we benefit from hydrating with water, especially at this stage in our lives. From the perimenopause onwards, the body feels as if it is effectively 'drying out', so keeping up a healthy liquid intake is essential. Current advice recommends drinking about eight 200ml glasses a day – that's about 1.6 litres.

Gynaecologist Jullien Brady explains: 'The whole-body effect of declining oestrogen levels is hard to describe or imagine. Oestrogen plays such a crucial role and its decline often leads to a feeling of the whole body drying up. Skin and hair feels less elastic, damaging more easily and certainly harder to maintain. Vaginal dryness is a problem too but also a dry mouth is especially common.'

My own rule is to sip pure, still water throughout the day, mostly between meals, so as not to dilute the gastric juices required for digestion. Although I take issue with the plastic waste created by single-use water bottles, I prefer not to drink chlorinated tap water. My solution is to use a filter jug at home and carry a portable water filter bottle around with me for on-the-spot rehydration.

Not only does water keep skin looking plump and aid concentration, it also relieves fatigue and headaches, and can help stop energy levels from dipping later in the day. Proper hydration in the early evening can also help you to fall asleep as well as enjoy a better quality of sleep.

Keeping topped up with water is essential if you travel regularly for work or pleasure as dehydration may increase the risk of deep vein thrombosis (DVT). Dehydration causes the blood to thicken, which means the heart has to pump harder to deliver blood around the body. This dehydration increases the risk of a blood clot, and therefore DVT, especially if you remain sitting in cramped conditions for long flights, or train and car journeys.

The caffeine connection

During the perimenopause you may notice your sensitivity to caffeine increases as it exacerbates mood swings from high to low. It is said that this everyday herbal stimulant spikes blood sugar levels, which can make us feel wonderful initially, but after a short while leaves us anxious and zapped of energy. As caffeine also works as a vasodilator – which means it causes blood vessels to dilate – we may sweat more and this in turn may trigger a hot flush if you're prone to them.

Nutritionist Dr Marilyn Glenville, who specialises in women's health, explains that when we consume any food or drink that has a stimulant effect, like tea, coffee, sugar and chocolate, its digestion is very fast, resulting in glucose entering the bloodstream too rapidly. This sharp rise in blood glucose produces a momentary high but afterwards we feel tired and drained, so we are more likely to reach for another snack or drink to give us a boost. As our blood sugar levels then peak and trough, so too do our eating patterns, leaving us with cravings for sweet foods and drinks.

Caffeine in coffee, dark chocolate, black tea, green tea and fizzy drinks works as a diuretic and therefore dehydrates the body (and we can lose important minerals and vitamins this way), plus it increases the flow of toxins and waste matter passing through the liver, placing it under an additional daily strain.

I love my coffee, so I enjoy making a ritual out of one delicious, freshly brewed cupful after breakfast, but try to limit it to just that. Certainly, taking any form of caffeine later than 2 p.m. can interfere with our ability to sleep as it stays in the system for up to eight hours.

Decaffeinated coffee is a better alternative, although take care to ensure you choose the water-extracted kind (as opposed to the solvent-extracted variety), as these contain fewer traces of chemicals which can contribute to the liver's toxic load. You might like to try red rooibos (redbush) tea, which is completely caffeine-free and rich in helpful trace elements and minerals, including iron, calcium, potassium, copper, manganese, zinc and magnesium. In South Africa, where most of it is grown, it's drunk with a dash of milk and sometimes a taste of honey.

What to eat in perimenopause

I've devoted much of my working life to exploring the healthiest and most natural options in the world of beauty and wellbeing, so it didn't come as much of a surprise to me that eating a good diet is crucial in the perimenopause. Nutritionists and dieticians alike agree that women should enrich their diet as soon as the perimenopause makes itself known and preferably *before* symptoms start, in order to help balance hormones which in turn will boost mood, sleep, libido and energy levels.

As the body undergoes this tremendous period of hormonal adjustment, it's more important than ever to nourish it properly with a healthy, balanced diet and remove as many of the modern stressors as possible. It should go without saying that a diet free from refined, overprocessed foods, damaged/hydrogenated fats, white goods (refined sugars/white bread/white pasta/white rice), artificial colourings, synthetic flavourings and excess salt is a good starting point.

Protein

The menopause is associated with a natural decline in oestrogen, which increases visceral fat mass, decreases bone mass density, muscle mass and strength. Muscle accounts for around 36 per cent of female body weight, so it's essential to increase the amount of protein we eat, which in turn can help prevent muscle loss and control appetite and blood sugar levels. It's easy enough to include high-quality protein at each meal as there are so many rich sources, from chickpeas, lentils, eggs and yoghurt if I'm in a veggie mood, to sustainable fish, organic chicken and turkey otherwise. Organic meats are important here as they are produced without routine use of growth promoters (a problem outside the UK) and anti-biotics in animal feeds.

Fibre

An unfortunate symptom of the perimenopause that can creep up on all of us is an increased appetite and cravings. One tip to help combat these is to include the recommended 21 grams per day of fibre. I'm a big fan of colourful vegetables and fruit, wholegrains and beans. Make your plate as colourful as possible – literally eating the rainbow of shades in natural, seasonal produce. Some of my favourite recipes here include Tempeh Wraps on page 141 and Quick Fix Kedgeree on page 189.

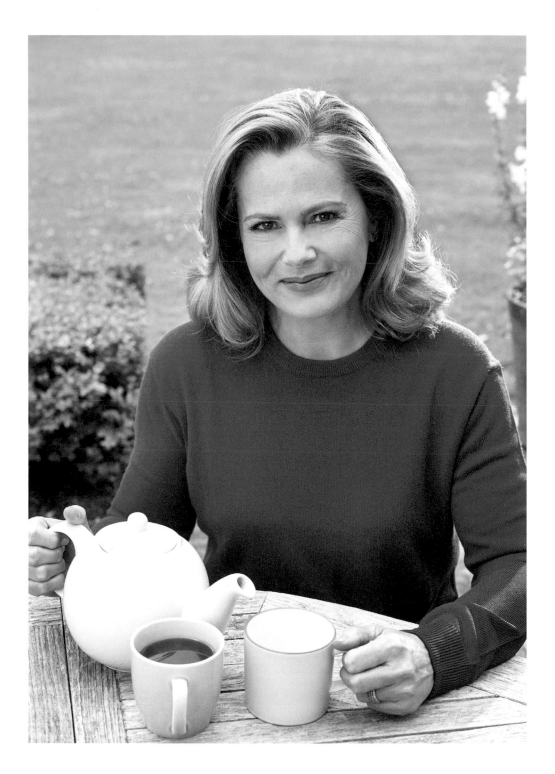

Vitamin D

To compensate for bone density loss, which is practically unavoidable as time goes by due to lower levels of oestrogen, pay very special attention to the two main nutrients associated with bone health and make sure you get plenty of them: calcium and vitamin D.

Vitamin D is so very important for calcium absorption and a healthy immune system. Good sources of vitamin D are oily fish, organic eggs, red meat (better to eat high-quality, locally reared, grass-fed red meat occasionally than to eat cheaper factory-farmed red meat more often) and foods fortified with vitamin D by the manufacturer, such as some breakfast cereals and dairy products.

However, it's difficult to obtain the required daily levels of vitamin D with food alone. We also need to spend time in the sun to make our own vitamin D – and the amount of time most of us spend outside in the summer sun (without necessarily being covered in sunscreen or clothing) is not enough. For this reason, the government has issued guidelines recommending we take vitamin D supplements during the winter months – 10mcg per day is enough for most of us, but it's worth discussing this with your doctor, particularly if you or they think you may be at risk of osteoporosis.

Calcium

While dairy products, egg yolks, kale, spinach, cabbage and sesame seeds are all excellent sources, it's pretty easy these days to buy food and drink fortified with calcium, such as breakfast cereals, mineral water and juices. Unless you're sure you're eating plenty of calcium on a daily basis, I also advise taking a good-quality calcium supplement of 1,200mg every day to help maintain bone health during the perimenopause and beyond.

Shun sugar

Tempting though it may be to reach for an afternoon biscuit – or even something 'healthy', albeit high in natural sugars, such as honey on an oatcake – this will trigger a sharp rise in blood glucose levels followed by a rapid drop. During the perimenopause, fluctuating sugar levels lead the body to convert excess energy into fat, which in the long term will raise the risk of type 2 diabetes and CVD. I prefer to keep Meno-tea loaf and Chocolate coconut pots – see recipes on pages 209 and 210 – on hand to help satisfy my teatime tastebuds. Otherwise, if I'm not at home, I keep a small bag of whole almonds (high in protein and vitamin E) or walnuts (full of beneficial Omega-3s) and fresh fruit with me to help restore flagging energy in a more balanced and sustained way.

The sad truth is that we need fewer calories as we get older, so keeping well hydrated, reducing refined sugar intake and eating wholemeal flour and pasta, brown rice and porridge all helps to keep us feeling fuller for longer and make us less likely to reach for sugary snacks in between meals. Eating off a smaller plate is a simple but surprisingly effective trick that can fool the brain into being satisfied with eating less. And interestingly, since drinking the probiotic wonder-drink kefir on an almost daily basis, I've found my sugar cravings have all but disappeared.

Face the fats

I've been an advocate of full-fat, whole and healthy fats for almost thirty years (since my very first book, *Vital Oils*, was published in 1991) and, thankfully, the trend for eating low-fat is finally abating. Healthy fats are especially important during the menopause as hormones are made from cholesterol.

Omega-3s not only provide anti-inflammatory benefits, but also ensure hormones are being produced properly, and they've been linked to decreased depression, improved brain and heart health, keeping the skin plump and smooth and even helping with bladder infections and vaginal dryness.

One of the Omega-3s, known as DHA, has also been linked to the slowing of Alzheimer's disease, so it really is well worth introducing more of the high-quality, 'good' fats into your diet if you haven't done so already. Avocados, oily fish such as salmon, mackerel, herring and sardines, nuts (and their respective nut butters) and seeds such as chia and flax seed (linseed) are all good sources. I also recommend taking a daily Omega-3 fish oil supplement to help boost brain, body and skin, especially during these, our more mature years.

B vitamins

Keeping up your B vitamins will also help fight against the risk of Alzheimer's, as they drive key processes in the brain such as methylation, which is needed to produce mood-boosting serotonin and adrenaline. The Swedish Karolinska Institute published a seven-year study of 271 Finnish people which found that those with low amounts of vitamin B12 (easily found in meat, fish, dairy and fortified cereals) were more likely to develop Alzheimer's.[8]

Weighty matters

If we want to combat one of the ugliest of menopausal symptoms, the dreaded night sweats, *before* they start, we need to be at our ideal weight. According to the latest research from the North American Menopause Society, hot flushes and the night sweats known as vasomotor symptoms (VMS) experienced during the menopause are associated with higher body mass index.

This supports the thermoregulatory theory which suggests that BMI is linked to VMS because body fat tissue acts as a strong heat insulator. The study also confirms other symptoms such as joint and muscular pain and urinary problems are more prevalent in those who are obese and, in some further studies, weight loss and exercise combined have been shown to reduce VMS.[9]

Those who have successfully managed an eating disorder earlier in life may find that the onset of symptoms in the perimenopause and menopause can trigger a recurrence. Medics don't have a definitive answer as to why this should happen, but believe it may be due to a hormonal imbalance and/or the loss of control over physical changes such as weight gain and a change of body shape beyond our usual control. Poor nutritional intake or purging can also raise levels of the stress hormone cortisol which in turn will accelerate bone loss, leading to an increased risk of developing osteopenia, the precursor to osteoporosis. It's also highly likely to trigger gut problems, such as leaky gut, acid reflux or IBS. If you suspect this might be an issue for you, do please seek medical help here sooner rather than later.

In a nutshell, maintaining a healthy weight and an active lifestyle becomes even more important during the perimenopausal phase of our life and will help ensure we stay healthy, happy and strong post menopause too. There's real evidence that the simple strategies I've outlined here can be of significant help with the many varied symptoms we may be just about to experience.

IN SUMMARY

- Check out family history to see if you are at risk of early menopause or any other health risks related to the menopause.

- Now is the time to take a good look at your diet and cut back on sugar, alcohol and caffeine, plus include supplements such as vitamin D and calcium.

- Monitor your body's changes and keep up regular health checks such as dentist, optician and audiologist.

CHAPTER TWO:
Symptoms

The perimenopause takes most of us by surprise – we may feel fabulous and in the peak of good health, only to become aware of niggling, troublesome changes, which when pieced together like a jigsaw puzzle suddenly make sense. One of my girlfriends visited her GP because she felt as though she was permanently about to come down with the flu, while another told me she woke every morning with stiff joints, feeling seventy-five and convinced she had an autoimmune disease. Being told by their doctors that they are not ill but heading towards the menopause was both revelatory and shocking in equal measure.

They join the 85 per cent of women who experience symptoms from the perimenopause onwards,[1] and, according to NICE (National Institute for Health and Care Excellence), 25 per cent suffer severe symptoms.

Symptoms of the menopause tend only to be felt while hormone levels are fluctuating. Be assured that these symptoms do not worsen and worsen for the rest of your life. Once the body has adjusted itself to a lack of hormones, the extreme symptoms often subside but can also continue until the end of our lives – another reason why we should consider some kind of hormone replacement strategy if we're one of those adversely affected.

I've taken a look at the worst of the symptoms below and hope the solutions will provide some relief. If there are fantastic solutions others would benefit from, do share – my social media details are at the back of the book. It's important to raise awareness in women who are 40+ and may consider themselves too young to be affected. Sadly, too many are mis-diagnosed with depression when they should be considering HRT instead.

SYMPTOMS OF THE PERIMENOPAUSE AND MENOPAUSE

There are simply dozens of symptoms associated with the perimenopause and menopause. Of course, those described below can be attributed to many other conditions, but whenever I've shown the list to friends, it's amazing how the penny suddenly drops for many of them!

Dry skin, weight gain, hot flushes, night sweats, sleep disruption, insomnia, exhaustion, mood swings, palpitations, chest pain, breathlessness, tinnitus, depression, anxiety, water retention, intolerance to alcohol/caffeine, hair loss or thinning, vaginal dryness, bladder weakness, incontinence, urinary tract infections, yeast infections, lack of libido, change of body shape, breast enlargement, dry eyes, dry mouth, itchy skin, hearing loss, memory loss, poor concentration, foggy thinking, aching joints, stiffness, gum disease.

Sleep disturbances

I've asked various doctors what their patients report as the worst symptom of the menopause and sleep disturbance wins hands down. For me, it was pretty much my only symptom and the one that sent me booking that doctor's appointment. As a busy working mother of five, I can handle most of what my life throws at me – but only if I get a good night's sleep. When that started to go, I sought professional help. However, most large studies don't show conclusive links between oestrogen decline and sleeplessness, so the picture is more nuanced than we might think.

For example, perimenopausal women, especially those who are obese, have a greater risk of waking up at night with a headache, which in turn impacts quality of sleep and may trigger more hot flushes, but science has yet to identify the primary symptom. What we do know is that, as oestrogen declines, the brain compensates for not receiving the hormone from the ovaries by triggering a surge in noradrenaline, which produces a fight-or-flight response in the body. This may mean suddenly waking up with heart palpitations, a burning sensation emanating from the chest and an overwhelming sense of panic, so dropping off again anytime soon becomes unlikely.

In perimenopause there is a link, according to a study, between poor sleep and where a woman is in her menstrual cycle. Research published in the Endocrine Society's *Journal of Clinical Endocrinology & Metabolism* found that women had a lower percentage of deep, or slow-wave, sleep in the days before a period, when progesterone levels were higher. They also woke up more frequently and had more arousals – brief interruptions in sleep lasting three to fifteen seconds – than in the days after their period.[2]

Rapid eye movement (REM) sleep is essential for memory processing, as is slow-wave sleep (non-REM), but healthy brain processing can only take place naturally – neither over-the-counter (OTC) products nor prescription drugs induce the same level of restorative sleep. As such, you may find that you have a more unsettled night's sleep during the perimenopause, and even if your sleep is not consciously affected you may feel more tired than normal during the day.

SOLUTIONS

1. **Follow sleep hygiene rules**

   Rules designed to help promote sleep sound dull but they really *can* make a difference. However, if they don't work after just a few nights I urge you to persevere for a whole cycle.

   - To avoid acid reflux or indigestion affecting sleep, don't eat within two hours of going to bed and avoid caffeine and refined sugars after 4 p.m. Check out your bacterial gut health too (see my previous book, *The Good Gut Guide*, for more on this).

   - Put down that screen, turn off the news or stop watching a movie one hour before bed. Exposure to blue light before sleeping suppresses melatonin, the hormone responsible for regulating our sleep cycle. If you simply can't resist one last glance at your messages before your head hits the pillow, stick a blue-light filter on your phone/ tablet screen. You'll find plenty of options online.

   - To enjoy a good night's sleep, it's essential to have a good day. Keep a notebook to hand throughout the day – use it not as a to-do list but to write down single lines of thoughts, be they anxiety-led or ones of gratitude, and review them at the end of the day. Considering how you feel as you journey through your day helps alleviate stress and the feeling that you haven't processed events as you turn out the light.

   - Spending some time outdoors, even if only for a fifteen-minute walk, during the day has been shown to improve quality of sleep during the night. Make sure you spend some time outside – even in poor weather.

   - Keep bedrooms clean, and clear of clutter and electrical devices. Studies show sleep is less restful in those with messy bedrooms.

   - Ensure air circulates and the room is not too hot – sleep with a window open if possible and ear plugs if needed.

   - Ever wondered why you sleep so well in a hotel with thick blackout curtains? The hypothalamus in the brain controls our internal body clock, which is set according to light signals received via the optic nerves. When light is registered, melatonin release is delayed and the hormone cortisol is produced, which raises body temperature and leads to waking up – so always keep the bedroom dark and cover up any annoying LED standby lights.

   - Eat thoughtfully so as to help your body ease into a good night's sleep.

2. **Meditation**

   Meditation is definitely an art but once mastered it can help guide you into a blissful state of mindfulness or contemplation. It's an effective way to mimic restful sleep even if you are not asleep, and if you are in deep enough you may then feel properly rested and be able to process memories. Look for a community class offering meditation, or check out one of the many new apps now available. My go-to app is Sleep Genius, which was designed using neurosensory algorithms to create sounds that guide the brain through the complete sleep cycle. It's based on research used by NASA to help astronauts sleep, and the relaxation and timed sleep programmes are both worth trying. When it's time to wake up, the app uses a gentle alarm to bring you out of meditation, nap, or night's sleep.

3. **HRT**

Hormone replacement therapy can make a hugely positive difference to sleep – see Chapter Three (page 40).

Hot flushes and night sweats

You may be spared some of the lesser-known symptoms (tinnitus, itchy skin, dry mouth) but three out of four of us will suffer from hot flushes and night sweats, making them the most common symptoms of the perimenopause and menopause. Few will escape the mortifying experience of trying to disguise extreme sweating/burning up/redness – which is all down to the hypothalamus malfunctioning, albeit temporarily.

It does make us sound a bit like a car breaking down, but decreasing levels of oestrogen affect the hypothalamus, which is responsible for setting body temperature, and it mistakenly senses the body is overheating. It immediately sends signals to blood vessels to vasodilate, which sends blood flow to the skin's surface instantly to cool it down quickly – hence the sudden, furious, flushing that pays no heed to whether we are at a lunch party, in the boardroom or in the theatre. The brain then registers its mistake so switches on the body's own sprinkler system in the form of perspiration to cool us down.

My girlfriends discussed experiencing everything from slight clamminess to rivers of sweat and those I have spoken to about this have always found it socially awkward. But so many women from mid-forties onwards have been there. They usually come on suddenly, spread throughout the body, chest, neck and face and can last a few minutes or longer, then vanish as quickly as they appeared. Hot flushes can be accompanied by dizziness, light-headedness and heart palpitations, which although unsettling are common and not serious.

Again, everyone's experiences are unique, so flushes may happen once or twice a day, throughout the day or one every hour. They can be triggered by eating hot, spicy food, or drinking alcohol, especially wine – and women who smoke are more likely to suffer more severe and frequent hot flushes.

Just for the record – as it's a common myth that always comes up – Japanese women do have hot flushes, although not as severe as those recorded in the West; but, unlike us, they do not have a fixed expression for them and their main symptom is of feeling hot-cheeked and dizzy. Research suggests that the lower incidence of vasomotor symptoms in Japanese women may be due to their high intake of soya, which prevents hot flushes. Edible beans, especially soya beans, contain the compounds genistein and daidzein, which are oestrogenic and so may help ease hot flushes. However, our differing gut bacteria means that this may not necessarily follow for Western women.

Although night sweats most often occur in the comfort of your own home, they're highly distressing and it's little wonder you're exhausted in the morning if you wake up drenched in sweat (sometimes several times a night) and need to change both nightwear and bed linen. One of my friends is awoken at 4 a.m. most days and likens the heat in her chest to a pizza oven; she can barely breathe and, after cooling down, feels exhausted but wide awake.

SOLUTIONS

1. **Yoga**

   A recent study from the University of California concluded that eight weekly ninety-minute yoga classes led to an average weekly drop in hot flushes of 30.8 per cent. While further investigation is required, this at least gives some hope that there is a form of exercise that might help ease the dreaded flushes.[3]

2. **Refresh and replenish**

   Avoid flushing triggers by stopping smoking and avoiding excess alcohol (or switch to vodka, a purer form of alcohol). Reduce or cut out caffeine and drink plenty of water to hydrate and refresh the body around the clock.

3. **Go natural in the bedroom**

- It's not easy for anyone sharing a bedroom to go through such disruption at night so one tip is to have separate single duvets and go for a lightweight summer duvet with a tog of between 3 and 4.5. Cotton or linen bedding is cooler than a cotton/polyester mix and allows the skin to breathe. Opt for low-thread-count cotton or, better still, long-lasting linen – which has a thread count of 80–150 and better wicking properties. When it comes to what to wear in bed, avoid synthetic fibres which don't allow the skin to breathe and wear cotton or silk which can be layered in cooler weather.

- Keep a facial tonic spritzer beside the bed, as the blissful mist evaporating on hot skin can bring instantly refreshing relief. Always take a jug of iced water to bed plus a small electric fan – which is most effective when switched on after a spritz during a hot flush. I've also been told about pillows with a cooling gel layer that provide relief, which may be worth a try if a burning head and neck are the issue. Alternatively, fill a hot water bottle with icy water.

Dull skin

As we head towards our fifties, it will be literally written on our faces whether we've followed a healthy lifestyle or not. And for all our best efforts to limit exposure to sun, wind and pollutants, the intricate role female hormones play with regard to the skin may not be so obvious. Oestrogen is key in building collagen, the protein that supports the skin's structure, so one of the first visible signs of the perimenopause is reduced skin elasticity. It can be subtle, but you may notice that skin looks less glowing, seems drier somehow and thinner, while volume from the cheeks heads down towards the jawline.

Helping the skin in its continual process of renewal are the blood vessels, fat cells, hair follicles and nerve endings. Necessary to all this activity are hormones and oxygen, delivered to skin cells by the circulation of the blood. However, as early as our mid-thirties, this hormonal activity begins to slow down – fat cells are reduced, collagen and elastin become weaker and the moisture content decreases, all of which contributes to skin wrinkling. Many women report acne – either for the first time or back with a vengeance – and increased facial hair, both due to hormone changes.

I always find it so encouraging that our skin grows even during older age, replacing itself every few weeks from its base dermal layer. It's to this that we need to pay the most attention and encourage stronger, healthier skin cells, through what we eat and drink.

SOLUTIONS

- Are you using the right beauty products? As we age, so our skin needs greater nourishment and nurturing, often with a richer moisturising cream, serums formulated for more mature skins and thicker body lotions, which are all likely to be soothing, comforting and a great morale booster. Look for formulations made with plants oils (such as cocoa or shea butter, rosehip, avocado and argan) which are better absorbed into the upper levels of the skin than the blander mineral oils that simply sit on the skin's surface.

- Good skin starts with good nutrition, especially as we age, so keep these delicious foods in mind when creating weekly menus and your skin can be better nourished. Vitamin E helps protect cell structures and membranes, so choose almonds, avocados, sweet potatoes, asparagus and spinach. Vitamin C protects cells and skin tissue and is essential for wound-healing, so think bright with oranges, red peppers, kale, Brussels sprouts, strawberries and broccoli. The mineral selenium helps protect cells and tissues from damage (including sun damage) and can be found in brazil nuts, sardines, yellowfin tuna, turkey, chicken and beef (especially grass-fed beef).

- To enable these nutrients to be absorbed and utilised effectively by the body, it's important to keep active and boost circulation by exercising regularly. When we do so, tiny arteries in the skin dilate, allowing more blood to reach the surface of the skin and deliver nutrients that repair damage from the sun and pollution. These also kick-start fibroblasts, the collagen-producing cells in the skin which decline as we age, and helps them work more effectively so that skin looks plumper and refreshed.

- Those I know who take HRT say it does wonders for their skin, making a swift and visible difference to sagging skin, improving both texture and tone, as well as minimising fine lines and wrinkles.

Hair loss and hirsutism

No woman over forty has the same volume of hair that they had in their twenties, according to my hairdresser, but none of us really notices the cumulative effects of this until the perimenopause, when thinning hair is difficult to counteract. Perhaps you first notice that gradually each strand is losing volume, is finer, weaker, less glossy, and you can't grow it as long as you once did. If you examine a photograph that's ten or more years old, you may discern a receding hairline at the front or temples, and actually just less hair altogether.

Oestrogen allows hair to thrive in a growing phase, and the longer this phase, the longer we are able to grow our hair, so it makes sense that dwindling levels of oestrogen result in a shorter growth cycle and the loss of hair before it reaches its optimal length.

Not only is our main female hormone receding, the menopause can trigger a rise in androgens, male hormones that exacerbate thinning of the hair, similar to the early stages of male pattern hair loss, while promoting excess facial and body hair. This facial hair can be in the form of a light or dark 'down' which covers the bottom half of the face and neck, or it may be the odd wiry hair which springs out from the chin or upper lip area, miraculously, it would seem, overnight.

SOLUTIONS

1. Hello, new hairstyle

Now is the perfect time to update a hairstyle that may have worked brilliantly before but needs a rethink, so discuss your concerns with a hairdresser – whether the issue is thinning hair or greys coming through. Clever cutting can disguise all manner of hair and scalp problems. Many find that a liberating short crop gives hair a new lease of life, and embrace their natural colour and the freedom from hair that needs blow-drying, styling and high maintenance. Of course, the reverse is also true and there are few easier or swifter ways to reverse the outward signs of ageing than covering grey hair with semi-permanent tints or soft blonde highlights woven between the grey (my own preferred method of disguise).

2. Lighting up

Avoid an 'Oh NO!' situation when returning from work or a social gathering only to discover a very visible wiry chin hair and invest in a well-lit magnifying mirror and super-strong bathroom lighting. Unflattering – but very necessary. As is keeping a good pair of tweezers permanently to hand so as to eliminate stray hairs as soon as they appear. There are also more long-lasting solutions to this problem, including laser treatment, IPL (intense pulsed light), waxing, depilatory cream, threading and electrolysis. All of these can be used to good effect around the upper lip, chin and lower jaw areas.

3. Vitamins and supplements

No matter how abundant or fine your hair, it will feed and thrive on a diet full of protein and essential vitamins, plus a daily dose of silica, biotin and kelp (seaweed) to further help strengthen it. You may feel your iron supplement days are almost over but the opposite is true – iron gives us energy, preventing anaemia and warding off feelings of fatigue, not to mention promoting better hair growth.

- Find much more on helpful solutions for skin and hair as we age in the chapter on beauty.

Aching bones and oestrogen

One of the earliest symptoms many women report in perimenopause is feeling stiff and achy first thing in the morning, with some slight swelling in the fingers, wrists and legs. Why? Oestrogen has a pivotal role in maintaining joint and bone health – so as hormone levels decline, inflammation around the joints increases. Dehydration can also trigger joint pain because an increase in uric acid may cause inflammation around the joints, so keep topped up with water. Daily stretching is also key to keeping joints supple and mobile.

Bladder problems

You may have had little or no experience of urinary tract infections (UTIs) or similar bladder-related issues – until the perimenopause. As oestrogen levels fall during the perimenopause and beyond, the smooth muscles of the bladder, vagina and urethra lose tone and, consequently, many women will experience an increase in pelvic pain, as well as a higher risk of bladder problems. The decrease in blood flow and lubrication to the bladder and vaginal tissue leaves them thinner, drier and more prone to inflammation, and renders it vulnerable to infection, which can result in symptoms such as a frequent, urgent need to urinate and a burning sensation, as well as light incontinence. In the perimenopause, you may experience cramping around ovulation or right before your periods and if you suffer from endometriosis or irritable bowel syndrome (IBS), you may have more pain from inflammation and scar tissue as your hormone levels fall.

SOLUTIONS

- Research shows that those with weakened back muscles may experience more pelvic pain, so Pilates, yoga, swimming and brisk walking at least five times a week for thirty minutes or more can help ease this.

- Avoid irritating the bladder with acidic drinks such as coffee, tea, fruit juices, tonic, soda, or sparkling mineral water (the pH balance of sparkling water is between 5 and 6, while still water is neutral at 7).

- Your first drink of the day on waking should be a glass of pure water, hot or cold, to rehydrate the body (especially if you've had any night sweats) and ease the bladder into action without irritation.

- Pelvic floor exercises are vital, whether you've delivered babies or not, and there are many regimes you can follow online – and even downloadable apps to remind and encourage you to 'squeeze' throughout the day to strengthen your pelvic floor.

Mood swings

Outbursts, mood swings, call them what you like, these are a classic sign of the perimenopause as hormones go through a state of flux and the body is constantly trying to balance itself and counteract the declining levels of progesterone. To compensate, the stress hormones adrenaline and cortisol are released, and it's these hormones that can increase feelings of anxiety, tension, weepiness, depression and irritability, no matter where you are in your monthly cycle. Progesterone acts as a natural sedative and is a calming influence on the body – yet supplies circulating the body during the perimenopause and menopause can drop to as little as 60 per cent. No wonder we can feel low.

SOLUTIONS

- NICE recommends cognitive behavioural therapy (CBT) be considered as a way to alleviate low mood or anxiety due to the menopause (see the chapter on emotions).

- Eat happy foods rich in Omega-3, such as salmon, tuna or mackerel – and bananas which are packed with potassium.

- Vitamin D is essential for healthy bones, teeth, muscles and our immune system, but some studies report an association between lower serum levels of vitamin D and symptoms of depression, according to Professor Martin Hewison of the University of Birmingham – although he warns it's unclear whether this is cause or consequence as those affected may not get outside enough when they are depressed.

- To help avoid spells of feeling in hormonal freefall, look to phytoestrogens such as flax seeds (linseeds), lentils, chickpeas, soya and green vegetables to help bolster mood. Research shows they help regulate hormone balance by mimicking oestrogen and may stimulate the liver to produce sex hormone-binding globulin (SHBG), which controls the levels of oestrogen and testosterone circulating in the blood.

Hellish headaches

Fluctuating hormone levels in the perimenopause can play havoc with your head, especially if you already suffer from headaches, hormonal headaches and migraines. When blood vessels in the brain repeatedly dilate then constrict, the result is a painful headache. During the perimenopause, they may be more intense, more frequent, closer together and bring with them nausea and vomiting. Take this as a sign that your hormone levels are in a state of flux, and be aware that knockout headaches will be exacerbated by stress, tiredness, erratic eating and dehydration.

SOLUTIONS

1. **Balance and energy**

- Eat small amounts regularly – every three to four hours during the day – and include protein and fibre to keep energy levels balanced.

- Hydration is absolutely key in helping to prevent headaches, dizziness and fatigue, so drink at least 1.5–2 litres daily, as headaches can often be a sign of simple dehydration.

2. **Brilliant breathing**

    Yoga breathing is excellent for helping to relieve stress and headaches – and a great technique to try if you don't want to take a painkiller.

- Sit quietly with eyes shut and for five minutes focus on slow, long breaths, counting to five on inhale and five on exhale. This will relax you and may reduce pain.

- Nadi Shodhana is a yoga relaxation technique whereby you inhale through the left nostril and exhale through the right, then swap over. This is not straightforward so make it easier by covering the 'resting' nostril.

- Bhastrika is a breathing exercise that helps prevent migraines and ease them, for some. Take ten quick, short breaths through the nose, filling the tummy and chest. After the ten breaths, take one slow, deep breath out.

3. **Massage**

    Massage is also very useful for helping to ease tension headaches, especially to help relax tightened muscles at the back of the neck and shoulders. Always take a break from sitting at a desk or from repetitive tasks, such as ironing, weeding or writing, to stand and stretch out. Fans of acupressure say this ancient form of healing – known as acupuncture without the needles, as it is based on touch alone – works wonders on headaches. When acupressure points on the body are stimulated, endorphins and oxytocin are triggered and work together to relieve pain, while blood flow is increased.

Vaginal dryness

Vaginal atrophy is among the very last menopause taboos, yet is one of the most common symptoms and directly linked to declining oestrogen levels. Not only does this make sex difficult and painful, it can also lead to localised skin irritation which in turn can trigger infection and recurring problems such as cystitis and thrush. Some women report conditions so painful they liken it to 'sitting on a bonfire'. For more on how it may affect sex and relationships, see the later chapter on that subject.

SOLUTIONS

- HRT will usually restore healthy body fluids within two to three months of taking it. For those who don't want to – or are unable to – take HRT treatments, a vaginal gel or slow-release pessaries or ring can be prescribed to help. Topical lubricants are also widely available – choose water-based formulations made without preservatives, which can irritate sensitive internal skin tissues. Three of the best brands are YES, Sylk and Regelle (available over the counter and on the NHS), made to the correct vaginal pH balance. There are also interesting hormone-free laser treatments available, such as MonaLisa Touch, which use a specific pain-free laser frequency to stimulate the collagen in the vaginal walls to rehydrate skin tissues and treat vulvovaginal atrophy. Although expensive and currently only available privately, these are reputedly highly effective at treating burning, itching and dryness in this most delicate area.

Weight gain

I'm loath to agree with findings from the International Menopause Society, who talk about 'The Menopause 10' and say women may put on a pound in weight a year – so if you start the perimenopause at, say, forty-five, you could be looking at a 10lb heavier version of yourself by the time you reach fifty-five. They claim that weight gain is a natural part of ageing, rather than being due to the menopause itself, and that the falling oestrogen levels cause the redistribution of body fat, so any excess weight gathers around the tummy rather than hips and thighs.

This is backed up by the Mayo Clinic, who add that hormonal changes alone don't necessarily cause menopause weight gain, rather genetics plus lifestyle play a huge role – which does make sense, as muscle mass typically diminishes with age, while fat increases and the metabolism slows too. They say that if our parents or other close relatives carry extra visceral fat around the tummy, we are likely to do the same.

In their book, *The Hormone Connection*, Gale Maleskey and Mary Kittel argue that whereas it used to take our body two hours to digest food, it now takes closer to four hours, allowing for greater absorption of carbohydrates, which prompts more production of the hormone insulin which stores fat.

Loss of muscle mass decreases the rate at which the body uses calories, which can make it more challenging to maintain a healthy weight, so of course if you continue to eat like a strapping twenty-something and don't increase physical activity, you are likely to pile on the pounds.

Research shows we need to eat 200 calories a day less than we did in our thirties just to maintain a steady weight. A simple switch to eating from a smaller plate and bowl can fool the brain into thinking we're tucking into a bigger plateful, trimming those 200 calories without really noticing.

One thing to be emphasised here is that during the perimenopause and into the menopause, the levels of exhaustion you may feel from time to time can be extreme, similar to the early days of pregnancy. The very idea of exercising when all you want to do is shut your eyes (not even nap!) may feel like yet another hormone hurdle to leap over, so it's easy to see how weight creeps up on all of us. Being aware of this can help spur you on and renew motivation.

SOLUTIONS

Move more!

- Of course, aerobic activity can help maintain a healthy weight, and strength training counts, too. As we gain muscle our body burns calories more efficiently – which makes it easier to control our weight. Consider taking up some form of weight lifting – either at a gym, or invest in a set of dumbbells for home use and follow an online guide.

- Moderate exercise, such as brisk walking for at least 150 minutes a week, is recommended by experts, or vigorous aerobic activity, such as jogging, for at least seventy-five minutes a week. I have friends who swear by golf, as this combines a tremendously long walk with the action of swinging a club – a brilliant move for maintaining a neater waist.

- Another reason for getting up and out is that women who do little or no exercise experience more severe menopause symptoms compared with those who are more active, according to a new study of more than 3,500 women living in Latin American cities.[4] They were asked about menopause symptoms, including hot flushes, irritability, sleep disturbances and depression. They were also asked how many times a week they engaged in at least thirty minutes of physical activity, such as walking, jogging, cycling or swimming.

- Researchers found that those who were sedentary (exercised fewer than three times a week) were 28 per cent more likely to report having severe menopause symptoms than those who exercised more. And another finding? Those sedentary women were also 52 per cent more likely to be obese.

Natural solutions to perimenopausal symptoms

While there is no hard-core medical evidence that complementary therapies work, anecdotally, women say there are a handful of herbs and supplements that may help ease symptoms of the perimenopause, and are also useful to have in your armoury when fighting PMS.

It is, of course, possible to have both at the same time and these natural solutions work wonders for some women, who see improvements in symptoms after the first month. To boost overall health, I recommend taking them alongside vitamin C and Omega-3 fish oils. Don't be tempted to 'top up' HRT by taking these herbs as well – they're both doing a similar job (although herbs are less effective than HRT) and if symptoms are still a problem while taking HRT then visit your doctor. Before choosing a herbal remedy, do make sure it holds a traditional herbal registration (THR). Any herbal products which have been approved by this system will carry a THR logo on the packaging.

Agnus castus may help balance hormones which can fluctuate enormously in the perimenopause and is recommended by some herbal practitioners for symptoms such as mood swings, tension and anxiety.

Black cohosh may help those experiencing irritability, vaginal dryness, palpitations, night sweats, mood swings and anxiety, as well as premenstrual migraines which may become more severe during the perimenopause. This herb does not have any oestrogen-like effects on the body, which is reassuring for anyone concerned about increasing the risk of hormone-related cancer based on family history. However, some preparations of black cohosh have been shown to be associated with liver failure.

Dong quai is used in traditional Chinese medicine and is recommended by some medical herbalists to help ease insomnia and sleep disturbed by hot flushes and night sweats.

Positive nutrition

If you suddenly find yourself feeling a little bloated, it can be tempting to go 'low fat', but I can't emphasise enough just how much the body needs good fats – especially now! Here's why: the body and the brain need fat to function properly, and we also need fats to absorb skin-friendly, fat-soluble vitamins such as A, D, E and K. Good fats include oils such as olive, rapeseed, avocado and nut, oily fish, nuts and seeds. Drink organic whole milk (preferably pasture-fed – look for the 'Free Range Dairy' label). Even full-fat milk is only 3.5 per cent fat so is not a high-fat food at all and is a rich source of both protein and bone-maintaining calcium.

A different scent

There's a subtle change that you may not have even noticed until I mention it; however, there are plenty of online forums devoted to women discussing a change in body odour – many complaining that, as they go through the perimenopause then the menopause, they smell different, they smell more strongly, they smell less feminine and they smell 'like men'. While many have suggested this is due to the increase in the male hormone testosterone, it is more likely to be as a result of the fading female hormone oestrogen. Your favourite perfume may start to smell differently on you too. Leave old favourites on the bathroom shelf and experiment with different scents. Explore lighter, fresher scents (especially citrusy notes of grapefruit and neroli) which, in my experience, can make you feel brighter and more youthful.

There are plenty of practical solutions to help ease symptoms, but it really is a question of trying different things at different times to balance how we feel physically and emotionally. I would always, always recommend that if you feel truly overwhelmed by symptoms, please see your GP – there is never any need to suffer in silence.

IN SUMMARY

- There are dozens of symptoms which you may be surprised to learn are linked to the perimenopause or menopause.

- For every problem, there's a solution – now is the time to try massage, meditation, yoga and to move about more to help with hellish headaches, anxiety, insomnia and weight gain.

- Many of us swear by HRT. Those who are unsure could try turning to herbal remedies in the first instance to possibly help ease symptoms such as night sweats, hot flushes and low libido.

CHAPTER THREE:
HRT

Hormone replacement therapy (HRT) remains one of the most controversial and hotly debated health topics of our generation, if only because it comes with a long list of benefits and also a few risks to consider.

Given the multiple conflicting studies that have been conducted since HRT was first introduced in the UK in 1965, I wanted to run through the latest advice, risks and benefits – and bust a few myths along the way.

At this point, I should declare my own views. After talking to many doctors and health professionals, not to mention friends who take HRT (some well into their seventies), it's obvious that even low doses of HRT can be of tremendous benefit and improve symptoms. I'm a big fan. As far as I'm concerned, HRT is simply topping up what my body is naturally lacking as I age and I thrive on it. Better sleep, smoother skin, improved mood and increased energy levels. For me, the improved quality of my everyday life, together with so many health benefits (which I'll detail in a moment), outweighs my own personal risk factor. And all this is freely available on the NHS – you do NOT need to go to a highly priced private clinic for so-called 'bio-identical' hormones.

That's not to say all women need to take HRT or all are suited to it. It's important that you discuss your own personal needs with your GP or specialist doctor, which will take into account family health history, underlying conditions and lifestyle.

What's in HRT?

HRT contains the oestrogen hormone to replace what our ovaries no longer make, or produce in declining levels during the perimenopause. Most standard UK and European HRT formulations are plant-derived from the oestrogen-rich yam plant and are body-identical.

Oestrogel and micronised progesterone, both commonly used in HRT, are derived from this tropical root vegetable. A substance called diosgenin, a precursor of progesterone, is also extracted from the yam plant.

It then undergoes several chemical reactions in order to become progesterone and is absolutely molecularly identical to the hormone produced by the body.

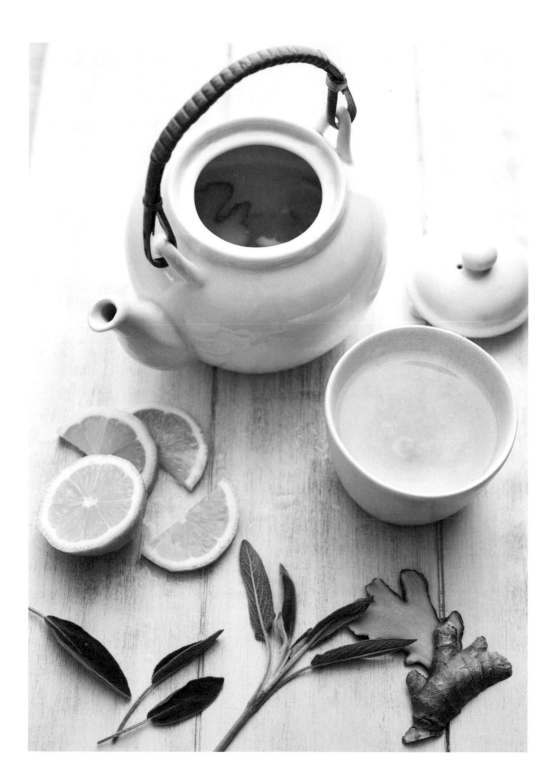

Some 'natural' progesterone creams are available online, but these are not recommended as they are not well absorbed into the body and may also contain too little of the hormone to be effective.

It's worth explaining here that you are likely to come across 'progestogens' which are a synthetic form of progesterone, originally developed because progesterone could not be absorbed orally.

How to take HRT

There are different ways of taking HRT and you can choose (along with advice from your doctor) the best one for you based on your medical history and lifestyle. It may be that you need to try different combinations before you find one that suits you. As with the contraceptive pill, there are plenty of different preparations of HRT and there is no advantage in waiting until your symptoms become really bad or even unbearable before starting treatment.

HRT is available as tablets, skin patches or gel – or even as a combination of these. The skin patches and gel are absorbed through the skin and are considered preferable to tablets, which need to be processed via the liver. Patches and gel are also recommended to women who are classified as obese.

Transdermal skin patches

These usually contain oestrogen only and come in various strengths. Some can be applied every three to four days and others once a week, and all of them work by slowly releasing the hormones, through a special carrier gel which is uniquely able to deliver ingredients through the skin.

Gel

This is unusually compatible with both lipids (oils) and water, making it more easily absorbed into the body through the epidermis. One or two pumps from the pack are usually applied each night. Oestrogen gel rubbed into the skin once a day has the advantage of enabling easy adjustment of the dosage – you might find you start with up to four pumpfuls as a younger woman, reducing to just one or two a day as you age. Young women with POI may actually need higher doses than this.

Tablets

HRT in tablet form is still the most popular method of delivery and it can be given as an oestrogen tablet for fourteen days followed by a combined oestrogen/progestogen tablet for the following fourteen days. It can also be given as oestrogen only (for example, for women who have had a hysterectomy) and also as a continuous type containing oestrogen and a progestogen. Consider taking the progesterone tablets last thing at night as they can help make you feel drowsy.

Progesterone can also be delivered directly through an intrauterine system (IUS) such as the Mirena coil, which releases levonorgestrel and works well for those who cannot take progestogen tablets. However, it is worth noting that the Mirena coil contains progestogen, which is not as body-identical as the progesterone derived from the wild yam plant which is found in micronised progesterone tablets.

Side effects of HRT

As with any new hormonal treatment, some side effects are possible in the first few weeks of taking it. The most common of these are breast enlargement and tenderness, abdominal bloating and fluid retention, irregular bleeding, nausea, leg cramps, indigestion and headaches.

The NHS advises speaking to your GP if you experience severe side effects or they continue for longer than three months. They may recommend changing how you take oestrogen, for example, going from a tablet to a patch, changing the specific medication you're taking or lowering the dose. Always take oestrogen tablets with food to help reduce nausea and indigestion, while regular exercise and stretching may help reduce leg cramps.

What about 'bio-identical' hormones?

For those who opt for pricier treatment at private clinics, an array of 'bio-identical' hormones may be offered as a supposedly superior alternative to an NHS prescription. However, these are very similar (if not identical) to most plant-derived HRT prescribed by GPs in the UK. They are deemed more natural than standard HRT – although the precise ingredients are unregulated so it's hard to be sure. In any case, natural does not always equal better (think snake venom, cyanide, arsenic etc). One thing is for certain: they are often eye-wateringly expensive, as bespoke prescriptions are created for each woman, and there are huge profits to be made from potentially vulnerable older women, who are often scared and ill-informed.

My issue with bio-identical hormones (aside from the potential profiteering) is that, unfortunately, they are neither regulated nor subject to independent medical quality control, so much more research is essential. Some women are led to believe that bio-identical hormones are in some way safer than regular HRT, but so far there is little scientific evidence to back this up. If you're tempted to try them, always check that any medication prescribed for you is NICE-approved.

HRT – the risks

Today, about one in ten menopausal women in Britain take HRT, less than half of those who took it a decade ago. This sharp decline can be traced back to research published in 2002, when the British Millennium Women Study published findings claiming that HRT raised the risk of breast cancer and presented a possible increased risk of heart disease. Understandably, many doctors immediately withdrew prescriptions, while the Medicines and Healthcare products Regulatory Agency (MHRA) issued new guidance recommending all women taking HRT be given the 'lowest effective dose to be used for the shortest time'. The reporting of this study was *not accurate*, but by then it was too late; many thousands of women stopped taking HRT overnight in the belief that the risks were too great compared to the benefits.

There are risks associated with HRT, the most obvious being that some types of HRT may cause a small increase in the risk of breast cancer. To put this into perspective, Cancer Research UK report that if 1,000 women started taking combined HRT aged 50 for five years, two more women would get breast cancer. This is a very tiny risk – and totally disproportionate to the scary headlines.

Breast cancer is frighteningly common. Each woman in the UK has a one in eight chance of developing breast cancer regardless of whether she takes HRT or not. Many are understandably concerned about knowingly putting themselves at an increased risk of cancer, but it is worth taking a closer look at the facts. The risk associated with taking HRT is similar to the increased risk of breast cancer in those who are obese, those who have never had children and those who drink two to three units of alcohol each day. Any increased risk of breast cancer with taking HRT is reversed on stopping HRT.

You may not be able to take HRT if you have a history of hormone-sensitive cancer, such as certain types of breast cancer. However, many of the findings concerning the increased risk of breast cancer are from studies that looked at women taking combined HRT orally rather than transdermally (through the skin in patches and gels).

Some senior specialists will prescribe HRT for women with a history of breast cancer, so if your menopausal symptoms are severe, it is worth asking for a GP referral to one of the NHS menopause clinics, or consulting a private specialist.

The length of time you take HRT for may also be an important factor. Most of the studies that look at the association between breast cancer and HRT have not shown an increased risk in women who take HRT for five years or less. Those who take combined HRT have an increased risk of having an abnormal mammogram, as HRT can increase the density of breast tissue. However, this is not the same as increasing the risk of breast cancer. It just means there may be a higher number of false-positive results that need further investigation to clear up.

Women who take HRT as tablets have a small increased risk of developing a blood clot or DVT. Again, the risk is more likely if you are overweight, have had a clot in the past or smoke. However, there's no increased risk of developing a blood clot if you use oestrogen as patches or gel, rather than tablets.

Some studies have shown that there is a small increased risk of stroke in those taking either oestrogen-only or the combined HRT. But again, there's no increased risk of this in women who use the patch or gel rather than the tablets. In addition, oral HRT containing lower doses of oestrogen seems to be associated with a lower risk of stroke compared to those containing higher doses, and most women under the age of sixty have a very low risk of stroke.

HRT in any form does not increase the risk of heart attack if started before sixty. In fact, taking HRT within ten years of the menopause lowers the risk of future heart disease, including heart attacks.

A large recent study, based on around 18 years of follow-up in 27,000 women, looked at overall death rates in women who took HRT versus those who took placebo, and found no difference. There was also no difference in death rates from heart disease or stroke, and no significant difference in death rates from cancer. This was the first study to look at long-term death rates among women taking HRT.

Cancer concerns

To date, there have been no studies showing there is an increased risk of dying from breast cancer in women who take HRT. Women who have had a hysterectomy and take oestrogen-only HRT do not have an increased risk of breast cancer. Nor is there any increased risk of breast cancer in women under the age of fifty-one who take any form of HRT.

The current official recommendation on HRT comes from Dr Heather Currie of the Royal College of Obstetricians and Gynaecologists (RCOG) and ex-chairwoman of the British Menopause Society (BMS), who says HRT remains an effective treatment for menopausal symptoms, particularly with the management of hot flushes.

Can all of us take HRT?

There are a few conditions and diseases where women should be prescribed transdermal oestrogen (instead of tablets) and these include kidney, or gall bladder disease, high blood pressure, heart disease, thrombosis, endometriosis, large fibroids, systemic lupus erythematosus, epilepsy and asthma. Those who get migraines *can* also take HRT but they should again be prescribed oestrogen as gels or patches rather than as tablets.

Testosterone talk

Testosterone is the third important hormone we need to consider when discussing HRT. Women naturally produce testosterone and this can be prescribed to work alongside oestrogen and progesterone. Our normal levels decline dramatically during the menopause as our ovaries stop working, which can seriously affect how we feel since testosterone helps boost mood, energy levels, concentration and libido. Even a very small amount of testosterone can have a positive effect on emotions and energy.

Low levels of testosterone are usually diagnosed by two blood tests: one for basic testosterone levels and another for SHBG (sex hormone-binding globulin), which assesses total bio-available testosterone and binds to two sex hormones – androgen and oestrogen. Its main production is in the liver, plus the brain, placenta, testes and uterus.

When levels of testosterone fall, sex not only becomes less appealing, but is not actually as enjoyable no matter how emotionally connected and physically attracted we are to our partner. Taking testosterone can help reverse this.

Again, it is a highly personal choice and not all women find it helpful; but for some, taking testosterone improves clarity of thinking. One of my friends says it's made her brain sharper than ever, and she's firing on all cylinders in the bedroom and the boardroom, while another came off it after six months as it made her argumentative when she used to barely raise her voice.

The crucial factor here is the dose: testosterone is prescribed as a blob of gel from small tubes or sachets (devised as one full dose a day for men) but for women there is no clear dosage. It's often left up to you (in discussion with your doctor) as to how much to use. The most common amount is about pea-sized. One friend who applies the gel daily says she knows she should scale back when she starts sprouting dark hairs on her chin! On the other hand, if she's heading away for a romantic break with her husband she rubs on a little more…

HRT benefits

Within a few weeks (even perhaps a few days) of taking HRT, the hot flushes and night sweats will usually subside and within months many women feel just like their old (younger) selves. Sleep, mood, concentration and energy improve and you may just feel happier – but then again, it's hard not to if aches and pains in the joints go and the texture of your skin and hair looks so much better.

From the first day of applying oestrogen gel, I slept so soundly, but other benefits can take a little longer to notice. Many women report their own moment of relief when they start to take HRT and it can vary from a few days to a few weeks. The greatest transformation comes within one to three months, with relief of symptoms relating to pelvic health, including a decrease in cystitis and UTIs and the frequency of needing to run to the loo. Vaginal dryness also diminishes, along with sexual discomfort.

There is good evidence that taking HRT within ten years of your menopause reduces your future risk of cardiovascular disease (heart attacks and strokes). The risk of a heart attack increases without the protective effects of oestrogen in the body.

Certainly, up until the age of sixty, the benefits of taking HRT usually far outweigh the risks. Oestrogen is pivotal in keeping our bones strong and healthy, so even if we take a low dose of HRT it reduces our risk of osteoporosis (see the chapter on bone health). Research shows that when taking HRT, there is a 35 per cent reduction in osteoporotic fractures of the hip and 34 per cent of the spine.

While this benefit is maintained during treatment, it does diminish when you stop taking HRT, although some research shows this reduction in risk of fracture stays with us for a time even after HRT is discontinued. In a review of studies, researchers concluded that HRT improved symptoms of oral discomfort, such as a dry mouth, in more than 50 per cent of patients, which makes sense as the menopause leads to a decrease in saliva as oestrogen receptors in the mouth receive less of the hormone. In fact, so many body fluids and moist tissues are improved, from dry eyes to the inner ear (reducing the risk of hearing loss and tinnitus), and the strengthening of collagen and elastin fibres leads to plumper skin. Oestrogen reduces inflammation in the joints, leading to a lower risk of osteo-arthritis, while testosterone has a positive effect on bone density and muscle mass. HRT can also really help with the low mood and psychological symptoms of the menopause.

10 GREAT HRT FACTS TO KNOW

1. Benefits are greatest for those who start using HRT within ten years of menopause.
2. HRT does not delay the menopause; it simply stops the symptoms while we go through it.
3. HRT is a daily treatment with *no cumulative effect*. The day we stop taking it, our body reverts to its natural hormone level at that moment in time and there are no ongoing benefits.
4. HRT does not cause weight gain.
5. HRT can lower cholesterol levels.
6. There is no link between oestrogen-only HRT and an increased risk of breast cancer.
7. Taking HRT does not increase the risk of cardiovascular disease (CVD) if you start taking it before sixty. In fact, it can protect against heart attacks and strokes.
8. HRT (orally or transdermally) does not increase the risk of developing type 2 diabetes and does not impact on blood glucose control.
9. Any increased risk of breast cancer returns to normal risk after you stop taking HRT.
10. Gradually reducing or immediately stopping HRT makes no difference to symptoms in the long term, although gradually reducing HRT may limit recurrence of symptoms in the short term.

Frequently asked questions

When should I start to take HRT?

There is discussion within the medical profession as to whether HRT should be used to 'prevent or repair'. Should we start taking it at the first signs of perimenopause to prevent a long list of health conditions and maintain a lustrous quality to our skin, hair and nails, not to mention preserve our mental health and avoid a potential emotional roller coaster? Or should we wait until our female hormones barely register in a blood test and we're actively seeking help for symptoms?

There's increasing evidence that the earlier HRT is started, the better the protection it gives from osteoporosis and heart disease. According to Dr Louise Newson GP, menopause expert and champion of HRT, we should not leave it until we're dragging our bodies out of bed each morning, giving the gym a miss and rowing with our partners. 'I wish women would look into HRT as soon as possible,' she says, 'and see it as a wonderful choice and a liberating alternative to suffering in silence with far too many dreadful symptoms which seriously affect our lifestyle and relationships.

'One of my patients started to take it and noticed a marked improvement in her skin – she had booked herself in for a facelift, a drastic measure but that's what she felt she needed to stop her looking so tired and old. But such was the effect of HRT that she cancelled the operation!'

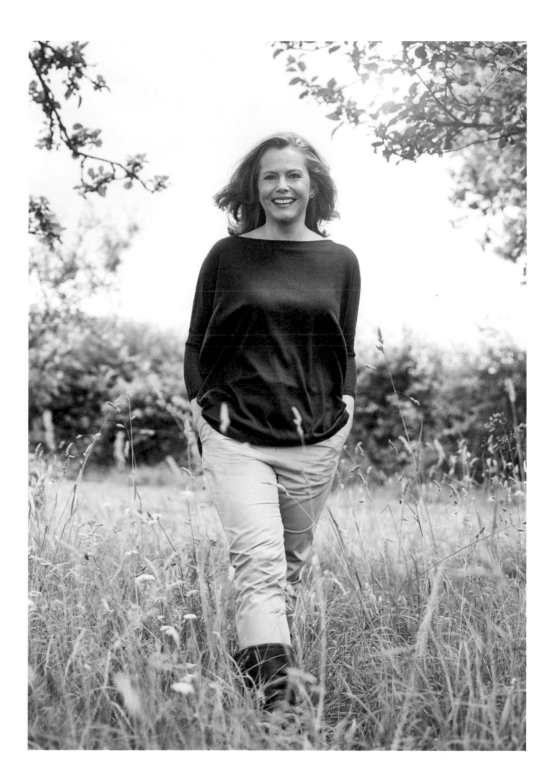

WHAT A COSMETIC SURGEON SEES

Olivier Amar, a French cosmetic surgeon at the Cadogan Clinic in London, says he can tell which women take HRT and which women do not just by examining the quality of their skin. While women who take HRT mainly want fillers and light rejuvenation procedures, menopausal women who do not take HRT are more inclined to request a facelift. And what do our French sisters make of HRT? They love it, *bien sûr*!

What if I am still having periods?

For those still having periods, a type of HRT that gives a monthly period will be prescribed and needs to be taken for around a year. It is common (and completely normal) to experience light bleeding or spotting in the first few months of use. You can start to take HRT if you feel the need even while you still have periods.

How long can I take HRT?

Menopause specialists do not recommend taking HRT for short-term treatment as this goes against all guidelines; however, there is no set length of time. Some take it for a few years to help improve the worst symptoms and, after this, many find their symptoms have disappeared. If your symptoms return when you stop taking HRT, this isn't a result of taking hormones but is because you would still be having symptoms of the menopause anyway. Many GPs are unaware that short-term use of HRT is not recommended. Many women in their 70s, 80s and even in their 90s still take HRT. There is no upper age limit for taking it.

What happens when I'm truly postmenopausal?

Some women decide to take HRT for much longer than a few years for its benefits of increased bone density and heart disease protection, as well as the improved condition of hair, skin and nails. Some women decide not to give it up because they feel better and have more energy when taking it – I have friends who are nearly seventy and say taking HRT is the best decision they've ever made. Dr Louise Newson's oldest HRT recipient is currently aged 92. But whatever your own decision, you should review taking HRT with your doctor annually and make sure you have all the attendant mammograms and other health checks appropriate for your age.

Will HRT help my memory?

There are studies that are neither recent nor conclusive which do suggest that postmenopausal women on HRT perform better in tests of cognitive skill than those who are not on oestrogen replacement. Several studies show the protective effect oestrogen has against the development of dementia, while one study suggests oestrogen enhances memory in those who already have Alzheimer's disease.[1] Still early days for global studies, but an important (some might even say *the* most important) potential benefit of all.

IN SUMMARY

- There are dozens of symptoms which you may be surprised to learn are linked to the perimenopause.

- The risks of taking HRT are probably lower than you may have been led to believe.

- Hormone replacement therapy generally uses the same body-identical hormones from plant sources (wild yams) that our body produces naturally. They are botanically-derived.

- Many of the niggles and health problems, large and small, that bother us right now may be due to falling oestrogen levels – which can so easily and instantly be topped up. '

- Don't be deterred by some GPs seeming lack of awareness around and reluctance to prescribe HRT. Do point out that NICE guidelines (by which all GPs operate) now confirm that the benefits of taking HRT outweigh the risks in almost all cases. A GP would not deny a diabetic insulin, so should not deny a menopausal woman in need of oestrogen.

CHAPTER FOUR:
Bone Health

It's such a shame that so many young women have little understanding of how diet affects their long-term health. But try telling a twenty-something that she needs to eat a well-balanced diet now otherwise she may well end up with crumbling bones when she is fifty-plus! This is why it's so important for young women to be discouraged from exclusion-eating (especially low-calcium eating, such as dairy-free) without a) good reasons and b) taking a long, hard look at the nutritional facts of where their high levels of absorbable bone-building calcium is coming from each and every day.

From our late twenties onwards, we can't build any more calcium into our bones, so it's a matter of bone maintenance – preserving what bone density we've got through diet and exercise. This is severely tested during the first five years of the menopause, when nearly 10 per cent of our bone mass is lost, while one in four women over the age of fifty is diagnosed with osteoporosis.

That's why I stress to my daughters (and please tell yours) the importance, whatever their age, of eating a well-balanced, healthy diet, which includes plenty of calcium and vitamin D, found in oily fish (mackerel, salmon, sardines), cheese, eggs, milk and other dairy products, orange juice and fortified cereals, plus rich plant proteins such as chickpeas and lentils.

I'm equally keen to encourage them to do weight-bearing exercise – an essential habit for life – as it helps strengthen bones and keep them strong. Weight-bearing exercises include any type of upright movement so pressure flows through the spine, pelvis and legs, whether walking, running, yoga, tennis or golf – all excellent activities for maintaining a healthy skeleton (swimming and cycling – though good for fitness – are not weight-bearing).

Remember, though, if you already have osteoporosis, no amount of exercise will help if you aren't eating a healthy, balanced diet.

It doesn't sound like a health crisis until we hear that hip fracture is the most common serious injury in later life, taking up 1.5 million hospital bed days in the UK each year at a NHS cost of £1 billion annually. Osteoporosis currently affects one in every two women over the age of fifty, with nearly 75 per cent of all hip fractures occurring in women in Western society. As for men, although they can develop osteoporosis, it is estimated to be six to eight times more common in women, who have a lower bone mass.

Osteoporosis

Osteoporosis, when bones lose strength and break more easily, is much more common as we age with loss of bone density occurring more rapidly in the years following menopause for women and continuing throughout later life. Loss of oestrogen plays an important part and the most popular way to prevent osteoporosis caused by falling oestrogen levels is to take HRT, as it's been shown to slow down, stop and even reverse bone loss after the menopause. It's recommended to be taken for a minimum of five years, after a natural menopause, to offer maximum prevention.

Osteoporosis is often called a silent disease because there are no symptoms until a fracture occurs or a vertebra collapses. If you've been unfortunate enough to be diagnosed with the disease then you're at an increased risk of fracturing a bone – sometimes with little or no trauma involved, such as a fall. So fragile has the skeleton become that normal activities such as sitting, standing, coughing or even hugging a partner can on occasion result in painful fractures in any bones, including the spine, hips and wrists. That's why osteoporosis must be taken seriously far earlier than it currently is, especially as there are so many simple ways to reduce the risk of developing the condition.

Calcium is critically important for maintaining bone strength. Calcium levels in the blood and bones are controlled by three hormones: the parathyroid hormone (PTH), calcitrol (or 1,25-dihydroxyvitamin D) and calcitonin. Our rate of absorption varies – so increases, for example, during pregnancy but decreases with a poor diet.

Calcitonin is a hormone produced within the thyroid gland, and preserves calcium in the bones by blocking the effects of PTH. Vitamin D is produced in our skin during exposure to the sun which must then be chemically converted in the liver and kidneys into an active form. The end substance stimulates calcium absorption in the intestine.

PTH released by the parathyroid glands also protects against low blood calcium levels by increasing activation of vitamin D by the kidneys. During the menopause, the kidney loses some ability to convert vitamin D into its active form so in the bid to keep a constant level of calcium in the blood there is a loss in bone quality and strength.

This is why eating plenty of calcium-rich foods (such as dairy products) on a *daily basis* is so important.

Weight-bearing exercise

Unless we have a back problem, we may never seek out specialist help from a qualified physio or osteopath, which is a shame as they often have a wealth of inspiring advice to give. Osteopath Nick Cowan is good at explaining why it is critical that we move – and that we move regularly. He says that as human beings we are designed for motion and this benefits us by improving the blood flow to our muscles and joints to maintain the health of our bones. As with muscles, bone

HIGH-IMPACT WEIGHT-BEARING EXERCISES

- **Dancing:** From tango to ballroom – these improve coordination and postural strength.

- **Plyometric aerobics:** Jumping or explosive movements improve strength and agility.

- **Hiking:** Walking over rough undulating terrain provides great stimulus to muscles (use supportive footwear and watch out for sprained ankles).

- **Jogging/running:** An excellent way to prevent bone damage – but do have your gait assessed and buy proper running shoes first.

- **Tennis/badminton:** The sudden change of direction during play means balance is a winner here.

LOW-IMPACT WEIGHT-BEARING EXERCISES

- **Elliptical trainer:** Low impact on the joints but requires high muscle stamina.

- **Floor-based aerobics:** With reduced impact but still emphasises muscle strength and balance.

- **Stair walking:** Testing strength and balance.

- **Walking:** If in doubt, always a good way to get moving!

- **Swimming:** With no impact at all but a degree of water resistance improves muscle strength.

is responsive to stimulus. Stress in the form of a load (or weight-bearing) stimulates calcium uptake and new bone formation. Exercise also promotes stronger muscles and enhances coordination and balance, thus reducing the risk of falling and possibly fracturing a bone.

'When it comes to exercise, it is important to consider your start point,' says Nick. 'If you've rarely or never exercised, it's never too late to start. For those already experienced, risk of osteoporosis does not signal calling time on a perceived riskier exercise. It's all down to gauging your risk through appropriate assessment and increased variety to avoid repetitive strain and overuse injuries.'

Here are his top exercise recommendations and how they might help us. I'm a big fan of walking outdoors every single day (all weathers – no excuses!) and at speed to get my entire body moving and energised. It's a wonderful way of clearing my head, especially first thing in the morning or after dinner to help with digestion and in turn aid sleep that night.

Nick also recommends lifting weights and using elastic/resistance exercise bands (perfect for packing in a suitcase if you travel a lot) as other excellent ways to stimulate muscle strength and improve balance and coordination. He also cites Tai Chi or Pilates as ideal for triggering those much-needed responses in the bone and muscle tissue, and helping to maintain good health and mobility in the musculoskeletal structure as a whole.

Nick's non-negotiables

Nick offers non-negotiables to any patient who visits his clinic and they are worth following – whatever your age!

- Don't sit down for longer than ten minutes. Any longer leaves you with a compressed spine and stiff shoulders, hips and knees (I'm now considering a standing-style desk).

- Do get up as often as possible. Your circulation will thank you and much-needed oxygen will flow through the blood.

- Do move your arms above the head. Start with shoulder shrugs, a Mexican wave, and while waiting for the kettle to boil get those arms swinging.

- Don't be afraid of the cold. The humble cold shower can provide a much-needed cardiovascular stimulus, boosting the immune system.

- Keep muscles warm. This may seem to contradict the previous advice but, while the cold benefits are true, intermittent use of heat packs, saunas, etc can provide heat stimuli to improve muscular function and increase blood flow to the brain. We are warm-blooded animals, after all!

- Try to sleep at regulated times. A set sleep routine will provide more than just a healthy clear mind in the morning. That vital time of repair at night is healing torn muscles, inflamed joints and all-round stresses and strain.

Am I at risk?

While being deficient in oestrogen is one of the most important risk factors in the development of osteoporosis after the onset of the menopause, there are others to bear in mind. There is a slightly higher risk if you are Caucasian or Asian, and an increased risk if you're fine-boned, underweight, vitamin deficient, have a diet low in calcium and high in phosphates (e.g. from fizzy drinks), drink too much alcohol and caffeine, smoke, don't exercise and, finally, have a family history of the condition.

If this has left you feeling concerned about your bone density, it would be a good idea to have a bone mineral density test or DEXA (dual-energy X-ray absorptiometry) scan, especially if you need a hysterectomy, as then you can see how strong your bones are and the results can be used as a baseline for later tests. If you choose not to go down the HRT route and you have a family history of osteoporosis or a history of eating disorders, then I'd recommend you consider booking a regular test to measure bone density every few years or so to help evaluate and monitor your bone health.

Facial osteoporosis

I'm fascinated by the approach US gynaecologist Dr Rebecca Booth, author of *The Venus Week*, takes with osteoporosis. When she wants patients to take the risk of it seriously, she just tells them osteoporosis will affect their face too. 'They are usually shocked and think it only affects the larger bones in the skeleton such as the spine, hips and legs – but not the face,' explains Dr Booth. It makes sense, of course, that our facial bones between the ages of forty and sixty-five look very different to facial bones at twenty to forty, and those bones lose density and volume at the same time as other bones, which in some women begins as early as twenty-seven. And bone density is strongly tied to collagen content, so a bone density test can be said to roughly reflect a body's collagen – interesting.

No surprises that it's oestrogen that has a powerful role in the promotion of collagen. Men, meanwhile, have a very gradual decline in testosterone (also a collagen supporter) because their reproductive organs do not retire, and this helps them maintain their bone density and muscle strength – they even experience less wrinkling compared to women at the same age.

'The orbital bone, that encircles our eyes, is a central feature of the face, and as bone density declines with the ageing process, our orbits widen a bit, causing our eyes to sink ever so slightly,' says Dr Booth, 'resulting in dark shadows and a loss of volume below the eyes. We focus on the wrinkles, but the framework of the bone is vital to support our skin.'

Protecting jaw bones and teeth

Far too many women don't recognise some of their symptoms as being connected with the menopause and oral health is a serious area of concern. There can be quite dramatic changes even if you have no history of dental issues. As oestrogen levels decrease, bones weaken and there may be bone loss in the jaw. A 2006 American Dental Association report noted that postmenopausal women with osteoporosis needed new dentures more often after fifty than those without osteoporosis.

Oral discomfort

Common symptoms often reported to dentists are sore mouth, burning sensations, altered taste perception and a dry mouth. One reason for this is that there are oestrogen receptors in the mouth and when the hormone declines, not as much saliva is produced. Yet another excellent reason to keep hydrated and to make sure you always have a jug of filtered tap water to hand.

Receding gums

Inflammation and declining hormone levels make gums more sensitive and prone to recession, which leaves teeth more vulnerable to decay. Bleeding gums are a cause for concern as it may be a sign of gingivitis, so do see a dental hygienist or dentist, who will advise on how to prevent further deterioration. Drinking the fermented super-yoghurt drink kefir (a very rich source of beneficial bacteria) has also been shown to help maintain healthy gums.

Tooth loss

Studies have shown that overall body bone loss may contribute to tooth loss in otherwise healthy mouths, which is a great incentive to crank up your dental hygiene by brushing teeth twice a day and flossing once a day, plus visiting the dentist twice a year and seeing the hygienist. One US study showed that women on HRT were 24 per cent less likely to suffer a loss of teeth, which is encouraging news!

How can HRT help my oral health?

Dentist Richard Marques is a fan of HRT if only because of its benefits for oral health, and he explains that the menopause may cause problems with our teeth and gums because of the drying effects of oestrogen decrease. When the mouth is dry, bacteria can grow, causing tooth decay and dental erosion (wear of the enamel), and it can make gums bleed or recede. HRT helps level out oestrogen and progesterone levels, meaning that dental and gum health will improve. For those concerned about oral health, studies have shown that HRT improved oral discomfort symptoms in more than 50 per cent of patients.[1]

However, some studies have shown that women who take HRT are generally more health conscious and one group had received more dental work and reported more frequent dental appointments. A Japanese study of 330 postmenopausal women showed oestrogen may promote tooth retention by strengthening the periodontal area surrounding teeth – without increasing oral bone height and decreasing oral bone porosity. The research concluded that there was a strong link between length of taking oestrogen and the number of remaining teeth.

Nutritional bone boosters and bone breakers

It's easy to feel confused about what is good to eat for our bones and what may have a more negative impact, but scientists seem to agree that protein is as essential as calcium and vitamin D for bone health and osteoporosis prevention.[2] That's because protein makes up around half of the volume of bone and about one-third of its mass, which is constantly being rebuilt. However, the same studies say it is important not to eat a diet too high in protein and that plant proteins, such as chickpeas, peas and lentils, are just as useful to bones as animal proteins, such as eggs, milk, plain live yoghurt and cheese (although their calcium levels are lower). Look out for foods such as breakfast cereals and bread that have been fortified with vitamin D, and only buy dairy milk substitutes such as rice, almond or soya milk that have been specially fortified with vitamin D as every little helps when it comes to bone maintenance.

There are some less obvious choices packed with calcium too, such as almonds and walnuts – and eating six or seven a day will not only help keep sugar levels on an even keel, but will also provide protein while helping bones. Brown rice is a big hitter on the calcium front, too, so is worth considering instead of pasta or potatoes for a meal. I use it in several of my recipes in this book and I particularly like the organic, short-grain varieties.

Oily fish such as mackerel, tuna, whitebait, salmon, sardines and pilchards are excellent sources of calcium (and canned are just as nutrient-rich as fresh) – just be sure to eat the bones of the smaller fish. It's the strong-flavoured dark vegetables that are the best bone builders, such as collard greens, seaweed, turnip greens, kale, okra, Chinese cabbage, broccoli and Brussels sprouts, but also soya beans. They're also rich in magnesium, while the mineral boron, which also helps maintain bone health, can be found in apples, pears, grapes, dates, raisins, strawberries, oranges, bananas, figs and pineapple.

I'm a big fan of beans for their high fibre and protein content but, unfortunately, although they contain calcium, they're also high in phytates which interfere with the body's ability to absorb the calcium from the beans. However, soaking beans in water overnight then cooking in fresh water will reduce these phytate levels.

Like beans, wheat bran contains high levels of phytates which can prevent the body from absorbing calcium, and it also reduces the absorption of calcium from other foods eaten at the same time. It's worth bearing in mind that when you're tucking into wheat bran and milk (such as with a breakfast cereal), the body absorbs some, but not all, of the calcium from the milk. To help, I'd suggest taking calcium supplements a couple of hours before or after eating 100 per cent wheat bran.

As much as I would like to suggest that everyone should eat a bit more spinach, please don't count on it as a source of calcium. Why? It's high in oxalates (oxalic acid), which means the body can't easily absorb calcium from it. Other offenders include rhubarb and some beans. This is why spinach is not such a great source of iron either.

I think there are few things quite as delicious as gently smoked salmon and, of course, it's packed with skin- and brain-friendly Omega-3s, but eating food with a high concentration of sodium (salt) means the body loses calcium, which can contribute to bone loss. Aim to eat no more than 2,300mg of sodium a day, and if a food label lists sodium as 20 per cent or more it's too much!

Other calcium sappers include alcohol (which also interferes with vitamin D levels), so limit intake to no more than two drinks a day for the sake of your bones, if not your liver. Caffeine also limits calcium absorption and may contribute to bone loss if you drink more than three cups of coffee or strong tea a day.

The fortifier in the fridge

My fridge is always kept well stocked with plain live yoghurt, which is an excellent source of calcium, protein, vitamins B12 and D. Research has found that higher yoghurt consumption leads to increased bone density and a reduced risk of osteoporosis. Scientists tracked 4,310 Irish adults aged sixty-plus and found that regular yoghurt eaters had a 3–4 per cent increase in bone mineral density compared with non-yoghurt eaters, with women showing a 52 per cent lower risk of osteoporosis (and men 39 per cent). The main message about yoghurt, according to this research, is that it's a good source of micronutrients, vitamins B12 and D, calcium, as well as protein and probiotics (in the bio or 'live' versions), and it could be a combination of these things that produces the beneficial effect.[3]

Essential bone supplements

You may find that your healthy diet plus supplements already cover all your bone health needs, but it's worth checking exactly what you're taking to see if there are any key vitamins or minerals you're missing out on.

A word of caution before buying any herbal supplements: check it has a THR – traditional herbal registration. All UK herbal medicines must register with the Medicines and Healthcare products Regulatory Agency (MHRA), the governing body which also oversees over-the-counter (OTC) medicines. If a product is approved by the MHRA, it is awarded a THR stamp and must be sold only for the conditions for which it is registered.

- **Vitamin K:** According to the International Osteoporosis Foundation (IOF), low vitamin K levels lead to low bone density and an increased risk of fracture in the elderly. Sources include leafy green vegetables such as dark lettuces, spinach and cabbage, liver and some fermented cheeses and soya bean products.

- **Magnesium:** While magnesium deficiency is rare, this mineral plays a key role in forming bones. However, our ability to absorb it decreases with age. Excellent sources include green vegetables, nuts, seeds, unrefined grains and bananas.

- **Zinc:** The importance of this mineral could not be greater when it comes to bone tissue renewal and mineralisation. Lean organic red meat, poultry, wholegrain cereals and pulses all have an abundance of zinc.

- **B6, B12, plus folic acid:** Research shows that these three crucial vitamins play a role in changing homocysteine into other amino acids for use by the body, so it's possible they might have a protective effect against osteoporosis. Further research is needed to test whether supplementation with these B vitamins might actually help reduce fracture risk, too.

- **Vitamin A:** According to the IOF, vitamin A intake is an area of controversy, because high levels of it may have a negative effect on bones, liver and skin. It is, they say, hard to eat the recommended daily amount (sources include offal, dairy, egg yolks) and the vitamin A issue only becomes a problem when too much is taken via supplements. 'Further research is needed into the role of vitamin A in bone health, although many countries at present caution against taking a fish liver oil supplement and a multivitamin supplement at the same time, as this could lead to excessive intake of vitamin A.' Instead of cod liver oil, a safer option could be to take fish body oil supplements if you're concerned.

IN SUMMARY

- Strong bones are crucial for a healthy, active and long life. Prevention of osteoporosis can be tackled through diet, exercise and lifestyle.

- Don't forget that bone health affects ALL bones so imagine how the face and jaw are also affected – and can include tooth loss.

- Include bone boosters such as plain live yoghurt, leafy greens and red meat in your diet and avoid bone breakers such as caffeine, fizzy drinks and – surprisingly – spinach (due to its high levels of oxatic acid and phytates).

CHAPTER FIVE:
Beauty

Most of us will have whittled down our daily beauty routine to a matter of a few minutes, using a handful of trusted beauty products and make-up. Of course, you may be perfectly happy with the serums, beauty balms and nourishing moisturisers in your beauty armoury, but I truly believe the menopause is *the* perfect time to take a long, hard look at your entire approach to ageing and perhaps make self-care a greater priority.

For too long in the UK, there has been a tendency to consider beauty treatments and procedures as 'pampering', whereas in other European countries, such as France, women see caring for their physical self as an essential part of being female; as maintenance, not indulgence.

And why is now such a good time to focus on beauty? I don't think I've met a woman who is going through the perimenopause and menopause who hasn't felt a dip in confidence (and that's putting it mildly in some cases!) when confronted by the inevitability of their changing body and face as the reality of it stares back at them in the mirror. But it's not in my nature to embrace the negative. I prefer to celebrate how we look and consider taking advantage of the hundreds of products, possibly even procedures, available to help lift, tighten, brighten and make us glow, so we can better face the world and the future feeling positive and happier.

Sunscreen for EVERY day

I'm starting with sunscreen as this is one of my non-negotiables. You can devote time and money to other treatments but if your skin is already sun-damaged then the results will never be as good. You should think of UVA as 'ageing' rays: they can penetrate the skin much more deeply than UVB rays, and the damage they cause results in the skin ageing. As we get older, our skin has fewer melanocytes, cells that contain the pigment melanin which is released to protect us against harmful UV rays. That's why sunscreen for the face and neck is not just for the summer months – UVA rays are just as prevalent in winter. If you don't want to speed up the ageing process, wear an SPF50 on your face, neck and backs of hands. This is especially important if you're outside gardening, playing golf or tennis, or walking the dog, as the skin on your hands may be stretched taut around a

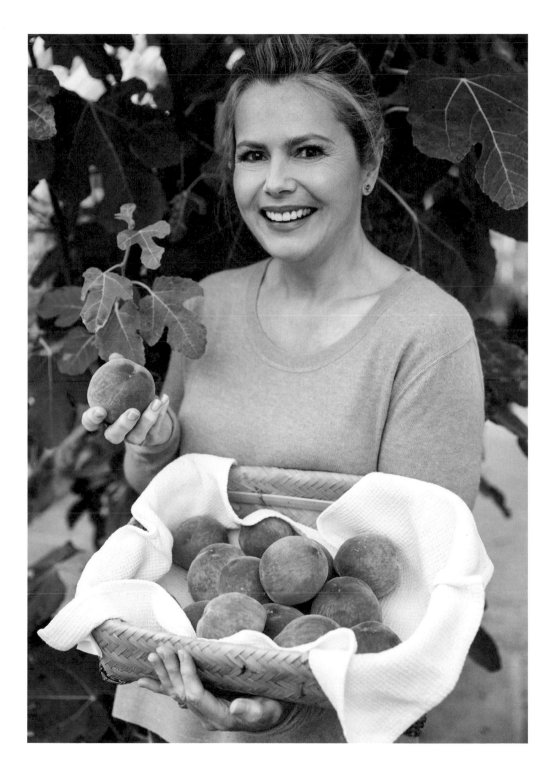

handle or lead, making it more vulnerable to the sun. Similarly, your right hand and arm if you drive with the car window open.

Moisturising is a must

I never change my tune on this one: for the most youthful-looking skin you need to feed your skin from the inside with a nourishing diet and then also be disciplined about a regular skincare regime – one of the most important parts of which is moisturising. The skin's ability to retain moisture reduces with age, so therefore it follows that the need for a good moisturiser increases.

Moisturiser smooths and protects the upper layers of the skin and helps slow the ageing process. It does this not by providing moisture per se, but by preventing trans-epidermal water loss (TEWL) by forming a film over the surface of the skin. It is this barrier that traps water within the epidermis to combat moisture loss.

Most of my favourite skincare ingredients come from the plant kingdom. Not only are they more often compatible with the skin than synthetic versions, they often contain skin-boosting ingredients such as naturally occurring antioxidants and anti-inflammatory compounds.

My go-to ingredients to look out for in moisturisers are plant (not mineral) oils – rosehip oil, avocado oil, vitamin E (from wheatgerm oil), argan oil, borage seed oil, shea butter and cacao oil. A good formulation should always sink in quickly and not leave your skin feeling sticky. I always look for those that combine plenty of skin-friendly ingredients such as essential fatty acids (EFAs) with vitamins and botanical extracts. A good rule of thumb is to look for the Latin botanical name on the ingredient listing, as this is an indication that the product has been carefully and knowledgeably formulated.

Slightly richer moisturisers are good for the dry skin that comes at our age and always apply to face, neck and décolletage (with a little rubbed into the backs of the hands for good measure). Then at night I prefer to add in an overnight serum or facial oil to give my skin an extra boost.

The beauty industry has woken up to the fact that older women would not only like to find enhanced products formulated specially for them, but they're also prepared to pay more for the privilege. Several newer skincare ranges are basing themselves around increased use of essential fatty acids and plant-derived phytoestrogens, as well as scientific breakthroughs such as EGF (epidermal growth factors) that may help skin better renew itself as we age.

Upgrade hand cream

It's still true that hands and neck are the biggest tell-tale signs of age, so I'm rigorous about using a rich hand cream after coming in contact with water and last thing at night. Again, avoid the mineral oil-based lotions now and go for richer creams with plant oils such as avocado or almond oil. Applying a generous layer of hand cream before slipping on a pair of cotton gloves overnight is a simple tip that really works to soften and hydrate hard-working hands. The same principle works with feet too: apply a good foot cream and wear cotton socks to bed.

Lighten up!

Concealers aren't just for our partied-out teens – we need them too! I usually find that puffiness around my eyes and any shadows dissipate within an hour or two of waking up (especially if encouraged with a little light fingertip massage around the orbital bone) but, if not, I use a brightening concealer containing light-reflecting microparticles. Pat a shade lighter than your natural skin tone into the inner corners of the under-eye area using the tip of your little finger. It's a good make-up artist's trick to help eyes look less tired.

Foundation

Tempting though it may be to apply foundation as thickly as moisturiser, it won't do us any favours. Think of thin layers instead – I prefer a subtler, translucent, barely there flicker of foundation to help create a naturally refreshed look. Invest in a magnifying mirror so that you can see precisely how and where to apply, and blend well from the chin down into the upper neck to avoid a tidemark. Once you find a foundation formula you like (and some of the newer, more expensive formulations are truly excellent), buy it in a couple of different shades so you can blend to perfectly match your own skin, mixing in a little more of the darker shade as needed during the summer months for a naturally sunny glow.

Buff up eyebrows

It will surely come as a huge relief that it's no longer necessary to devote so much time to hair removal (apart from certain specifics on the face …). But the flipside is that you may suddenly wake up to find that your once full brows look as if you've overdone it with the tweezers, and there are few things more ageing than spindly, sparse brows. If you're reading this in your early years, or talking to your daughters, the rule is: don't over-pluck.

To coax eyebrows back into life, here are a few tips which I've added into my daily beauty routine – but do have patience as regrowth won't happen overnight. I like to massage my dry scalp before washing my hair – always use the pads of fingers and not the nails – and this stimulates circulation and blood flow to the area which in turn encourages growth, and I do the same thing for my brows. Among its many beauty uses, coconut oil works as a basic brow conditioner and may help stimulate the roots if gently rubbed into the eyebrows every night. Massaging in a little avocado or olive oil works just as well, as long as it's done regularly (add a drop of lavender or neroli oil for a relaxing scent).

For a daily enhanced effect, invest in a matte eyeshadow the same colour as your brows and brush it through your eyebrows in short, upward strokes using a small eyeshadow brush, extending slightly at the ends to give the illusion of subtly fuller brows. Set your brows in place by combing through a dab of hair gel, or spray an old mascara brush with hairspray and comb through.

Look after lashes

Along with eyebrows and the very hair on our heads, lashes can of course become sparser too. Applying several layers of a lash-conditioning mascara is an effective way of boosting volume (try a deep, dark brown for a more natural look). Don't be tempted to try the eyelash 'regeneration' gels and serums, which as well as being very expensive have been found to trigger eye irritations and even cause eyelashes to fall out – the very thing they are supposed to prevent.

Another option is to have eyelashes dyed – it's a real boost to look quite awake in the mirror first thing. You can consider long-lasting eyelash extensions, which can be just the treat for holidays and special occasions and last a good few weeks. However, keep in mind that regular use leaves eyelashes weakened, and you may even find you lose some of your own along the way.

A safer alternative is to use lightweight strips of false eyelashes – buy the most natural-looking ones you can find and trim to fit. I find it flattering and more natural-looking to use a short strip just on the end of my eyelids, or even simply to boost my own natural lashes with a few individuals on the outer edges of the eyes. Just be sure never to pull them off as this weakens your natural lashes – remove by loosening the lash adhesive with a dab of plant oil or oily cleanser on a cotton bud.

Another trick to make lashes appear fuller and more lustrous is to apply a very dark brown or black eye liner pencil *inside* the rim of your upper eyelid. Sounds scary, but if you use a very soft waterproof eyeliner pencil, this is a great trick for thickening up the appearance of your lash line.

Thicker, fuller hair

You may be missing the days when you could simply wash and go, but as hair becomes finer, limper or coarser and drier, it may need a lot more love. It does pay off to upgrade your shampoo to a sulphate-free one that is less likely to irritate a sensitive scalp. Just make sure it says it will colour-protect hair if you have a tint or highlights, as some of the more 'natural' formulations can strip colour-treated hair. Only shampoo once when you do wash your hair – any more than this can overly dry the hair as well as the scalp, and will also fade colour faster.

The other essential for older tresses is to use a richer conditioner and/or a hair mask every week or so for deeper conditioning, to leave hair soft and silky smooth. And don't forget that heat dries and damages fine hair, so turn down the setting on your hairdryer and use a heat-protecting styling spray if using hair straighteners or tongs.

Greying hair is, of course, another biggie for so many of us. There seem to be two schools of thought here: either embrace our new grey/white hair or head for the hair dye. Personally, I don't feel ready to have my hair define my age to the world at large, so I prefer the latter. One of the reasons I am now blonder in my fifties is that my root regrowth is less obvious and my silvery grey strands blend more easily into the blonde. Others, with naturally darker hair, may prefer to tint their tresses back to their more youthful tones. A third option is to throw caution to the wind and embrace a full-on colour shift – witness the rise in pink, blue and purple hair hues. Now that's a statement, and it can be both empowering and very flattering too.

A word about 'down below' and the sensitive question of greying pubic hair. It's all very well asking your hairdresser to put the hair on your head into foils, but what about the nether regions? For those either still in or going back out into the dating world, patchy pubes can be a cause for concern. I was having this discussion over (a few) drinks with girlfriends not long ago and one announced that she found the greying so disconcerting that she'd had laser hair removal on the entire area (we gasped!). A less dramatic suggestion was the use of moustache dye, which I gather is both long-lasting and highly effective at restoring softness and curl, as well as colour.

Cosmetic treatments

There are literally millions of women trying to stop the ageing process in its tracks, so it's no surprise that the global medical aesthetics market is set to exceed £10 billion by the end of 2021. Women still account for 91 per cent of all cosmetic procedures – and 46,526 of them were carried out in the UK in 2015, a rise of 12.5 per cent from the previous year, according to the British Association of Aesthetic Plastic Surgeons (BAAPS). The most popular procedures remain breast augmentation followed by blepharoplasty (eyelid surgery), face/neck lift, breast reduction and liposuction.

Please always see consultants who are BAAPS-registered – even intelligent women have been known to have Botox administered by their dentist or hairdresser, which can be a mistake. If you do go down the cosmetic enhancement route, put your face in the hands of a properly trained medical practitioner experienced in clinical facial anatomy.

My own preference is to take the natural route first – but I then ask myself: what is natural? What if a treatment only uses a by-product of my body and reinjects it to stimulate what is already there? I've known friends feel tremendously low about their fading looks and seen them, after a cosmetic procedure, buoyed up, happy and much more positive about life, over something that might have been imperceptible to you or me, but seemed a real confidence killer to them.

One of my friends felt her earlobes had been stretched by years of wearing super-dangly earrings which she thought left her looking like an elder tribeswoman. She had them surgically reduced and was so thrilled with the results that she started wearing her hair up in a ponytail, which in turn made her look younger. For her, a simple procedure had a very positive outcome.

I'm all for doing something that makes you feel more confident and more alive. I became bothered by small age spots on my hands, and had them removed by laser which made me feel less self-conscious on TV and in photographs. My family had never noticed them, but I had – and I now prefer my hands without them.

Thankfully, the days of extreme cosmetic surgery are mostly gone and more natural refinement is the order of the day, with treatments that need little or no downtime, are not permanent and are incredibly subtle. It's often really hard to tell whether a friend has had a little procedural tweak, or has just come back from a relaxing holiday. For me, that is the best kind of 'work'. The treatments below are I think some of the better (if pricey) pick-me-ups and I would consider these ahead of any more extreme, permanent procedures involving lots of downtime. You may have heard about some of them before, but the constant new developments in the cosmetic industry mean better results can be expected than ten or even five years ago.

Hyaluronic acid

Its name sounds rather harsh, as if it might burn the skin, but hyaluronic acid (HA) forms naturally in the body, although supplies wane as we age. It's an incredibly strong substance and, as a humectant, it attracts water directly from the atmosphere and draws moisture to the skin so it appears plumper. It can also be injected directly into the skin to bolster the skin's own natural supplies, and studies show that it seems to stimulate our own HA and collagen reserves into renewed activity. Many popular cosmetic filler brands such as Juvéderm, Restylane, Emervel and Perlane contain HA for plumping out lips and filling in wrinkles. But we don't need to see a cosmetic surgeon to feel its benefits – HA is also a popular ingredient in plenty of serums available from high-end to high-street brands. You can also take hyaluronic acid as a skin supplement. My favourite is in liquid form and I add a spoonful to juices or smoothies, creating a skin-friendly 'shot' combined with another skin-saving supplement such as liquid or powdered collagen.

Facial skin peels

The good news is that the latest generation of skin peels can be used to refresh hands and neck as well as the face. Most clinics offer a programme of chemical treatments created to deeply exfoliate the skin and encourage the growth of new skin cells. This is not a one-off process and a course of treatments is recommended over six weeks or so, backed up with specialist skincare for maximum results. Facial peels these days are gentler than they sound, have no adverse side effects (aside from temporary reddening in some cases) and can significantly soften sun-damaged facial wrinkles, leaving skin feeling softer and looking smoother.

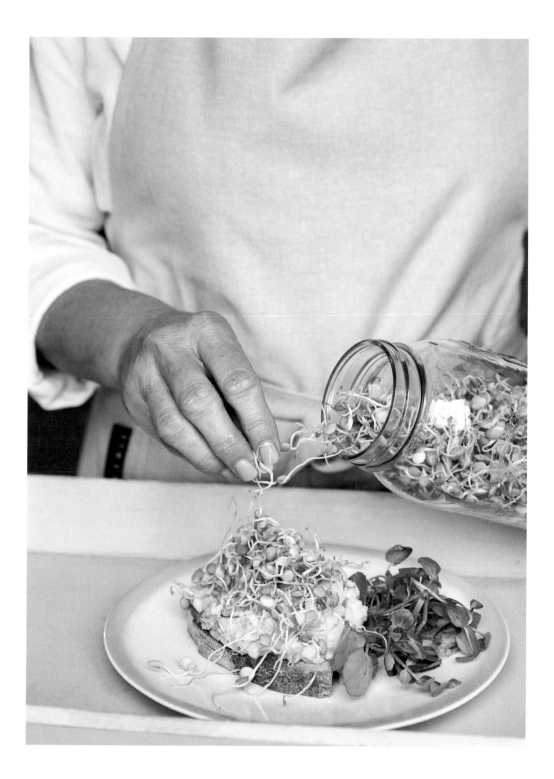

Microneedling

Well, it's 'organic', it's certainly self-repair and I'm told the tight sunburn feel and flushed look afterwards is worth it for the results. Microneedling uses tiny needles to make minute punctures all over the face, which triggers the body's wound-healing response. The skin repairs itself by producing new collagen and elastin fibres, which plump up the skin.

It's ideal to help combat scarring, enlarged pores, wrinkles, sun damage and age spots, but is not suitable for anyone with rosacea, psoriasis or eczema, or if you've had recent facial fillers. There's no risk of hyperpigmentation as the melanocytes and epidermis stay intact and the skin generally heals within twenty-four hours, although visible results can take around six to eight weeks to be noticeable.

PRP Express

One of the UK's leading cosmetic surgeons, Olivier Amar, is at the forefront of non-invasive 'anti-ageing' techniques and has created the PRP Express. It works by taking platelet-rich plasma (PRP) from the patient's blood. Rich in growth factors, the PRP is then injected through a tiny cannula into the cheek's deep tissue and this helps rejuvenate the skin by activating its own natural defences. This in turn produces collagen and healing platelet-rich plasma to heal the skin from the inside out. The 'express' part is so-called because the procedure takes around thirty minutes with no downtime and the effects are visible within ten days and last for six or so months. Friends who don't like the idea of synthetic fillers and prefer a natural solution say it leaves them with 'a just back from holiday glow'.

Laser skin resurfacing

Laser is now one of the most popular treatments for ageing skin and works by using thermal energy to remove the very outer layers of skin, encouraging new skin to grow. Always have a consultation before booking a procedure as the different sorts of laser – ablative laser therapy, non-ablative laser therapy, fractional laser therapy and photodynamic therapy – have very different benefits.

One of the least invasive treatments is ClearLift non-ablative skin resurfacing, which in around twenty minutes treats fine lines, wrinkles, small veins and redness. It is gentle enough to treat delicate skin around the eyes, neck, mouth and chest. As this laser heats deep beneath the skin (up to 3mm in depth) numbing is not required beforehand and skin healing occurs without damaging the outer layer of skin. You may need multiple treatments but this procedure does have the advantage of fewer complications.

Facial acupuncture

If needles don't bother you, then cosmetic facial acupuncture can be a wonderful way of stimulating the body's own cell regrowth. Acupuncture is a 2,000-year-old form of Chinese medicine in which fine needles are inserted into the skin at certain points on the body and is used to treat everything from backache and stomach problems to migraines and fertility problems. Fans say facial acupuncture reduces wrinkles, eliminates fine lines, lifts sagging skin and improves skin tone and texture, with effects lasting up to three months. Most practitioners recommend a course of ten sessions to see results and each one lasts around forty-five minutes.

The needles are inserted at pressure points corresponding to major organs so that energy and endorphins are released, and it's this minor trauma which improves blood flow, stimulates cell regrowth and helps the body rejuvenate. By traumatising our skin in this way, the production of collagen is stimulated, that very elusive protein which is starting to disappear from the menopausal body.

COLLAGEN BOOSTERS

To support the body's dwindling collagen production, eat foods rich in vitamin C, such as kale, spinach, citrus fruits and tomatoes, plus plenty of colourful fruit and veggies, such as beetroot, red peppers and broccoli as well as all the berries from strawberries and raspberries to blueberries and blackberries. For a real skin boost, try collagen powder, an increasingly popular skin supplement which can be scooped into smoothies, porridge, muesli, yoghurt – do bear in mind that most of it is bovine- or marine-derived so is not suitable for vegetarians. You may also be able to boost collagen supplies by eating foods rich in glycine and proline, two of the amino acids needed to create collagen. Studies show that some forms of bone broth may be helpful here (as well as good for overall gut health), notably chicken bone and beef bone broth.

Eye protection

As we age, excessive sun and wind exposure can see the whites of the eyes fade to yellow due to damage of the DNA in cells. To keep the whites of your eyes bright and protect the surrounding skin from sun damage, wear large-frame sunglasses with 100 per cent UV protection when outside in bright light. If your eyes have a tendency to redden or get dry in the heat or air-conditioned buildings then use saline drops to keep them looking fresh.

MY GO-TO REGIME FOR SUPER MENOPAUSE SKIN

We're now at a stage in our lives where we need to be really rigorous about our beauty regime if we're looking to minimise the inevitable signs of ageing. For me, this regime gives my ageing skin the best opportunity to look and feel clearer, smoother and well-rested.

EVERY DAY:

- Cleanse face with a foam-free cleanser, twice a day, every day.
- Moisturise with a plant-oil based cream, twice a day, every day.
- Add a serum into your daily routine, for both face and neck.
- Use a high-factor mineral-based sunscreen on face, neck and backs of the hands when outside, all year.
- Aim to have at least one mainly vegetable juice every day.
- Take nutritional supplements including natural-source vitamin E, vitamin D (may not be needed in the summer), calcium, fish oils and high-strength, multi-strain probiotics.

- Exercise – take a walk, stay active, every day.
- BREATHE! Remind yourself how to breathe properly and relax your shoulders.
- Be still – set aside a few minutes of quietness, meditation or prayer in the day to clear your head and calm your body.
- Enjoy a soothing bath or shower after dry skin body brushing. Always apply body cream after bathing.
- Sleep for seven or eight hours every night.
- Drink plenty of filtered water – 1.5–2 litres sipped throughout the day.
- Eat unprocessed foods with plenty of plant matter – green veggies and some fruit (I use the 70:30 ratio).

EVERY WEEK:

- Have a facial or a steam at home.
- Apply a face mask.

- Enjoy a home manicure.
- Enjoy a full-body scrub in the shower.

EVERY FORTNIGHT:

- Enjoy a home pedicure.

EVERY MONTH:

- Book a beauty treatment such as an all-over body massage or professional facial.

Beauty and the body

I know that many women find it much more of a challenge to maintain their physical shape (just to stay looking the same) once they hit the menopause, so it helps to know exactly what is going on – and to have a few solutions at hand.

Back fat and all that

We know that our hormones are inextricably linked to nearly all the changes that take place in the body after the age of forty. Until then excess fat tended to be carried on the hips and thighs, but not now. Fat storage shifts to the tummy and a new, unlovely area of podginess – back fat.

Falling levels of oestrogen trigger the body to use sugar and starches less efficiently; not only that, the lower our oestrogen levels, the more we tend to eat and the less we feel like moving too. To work and tone the upper back, try using a rowing machine and doing lateral raises with weights (invest in a set of dumbbells so you can do these at home).

You don't need to burn up at a gym (although that's fine too) to tackle the dreaded 'muffin top'. Yale University found that those with high levels of the stress hormone cortisol were more likely to carry fat around their tummies and have a muffin top spilling over their jeans. The antidote? Yoga! Those who practised it had lower stress levels than those women who did not. Swimming twice a week for twenty-four weeks also saw a 15 per cent reduction in body fat for women who took part – and an 8 per cent drop in blood pressure.

Breasts

Scientists at the University of California have found that breast tissue ages at a faster rate than any other body tissue in women after the age of forty-six. A mixture of hormones and gravity, plus the disappearance of fat and fibrous tissue, means our breasts will not look the same as they did before having children or in our thirties. Swimming, yoga, Pilates, push-ups and bench presses will help support the muscles beneath the breast tissue. This is an ideal time to have a bra fitting and to seek advice on how to get the best support and lift from your underwear.

Cosmetic surgeon Olivier Amar of the Cadogan Clinic performs what he calls a 'menopause makeover' for clients who feel their breasts have become too large, too heavy and are causing them back pain. He performs an uplift and reduction in breast size which helps women feel lighter, enjoy better posture and feel more positive about their changing bodies.

Perfect posture

We can usually guess the rough age of someone walking in front of us because of their gait and posture. It's a sad fact that, as they reach the menopause, most women walk more slowly and don't hold themselves upright – and 'tech neck' (double chin(s) and wrinkly neck caused by overuse of gadgets) gets to older folk too.

One of the easiest ways to knock years off how you look is to make a real effort to improve posture – and it is never too late to start. By standing truly upright, feet flat on the ground, head looking straight ahead, shoulders back and lowered, you immediately feel more alive, certainly taller, and it lifts the breasts. Take slow, deep breaths in and out and try to remember how this posture feels, so that you can recreate it when walking. Try to pick up the pace whenever out walking so that it is an effective form of exercise rather than just a means of getting somewhere. As you become more conscious of how you stand, sit and move then you will automatically start to correct yourself. I'm the first to admit that it's difficult to break old posture habits but I love this one tip for releasing tension and lowering shoulders: hold your arms behind your back and grasp the opposite elbow – this immediately brings you to a more upright position and you can feel the shoulders relaxing downwards. It's a great movement to hold while waiting for the kettle to boil or if taking a break from your desk or driving.

Pilates and yoga are two excellent disciplines for promoting great posture – and you don't need to be a bendy twenty-something to take them up. Two inspirational high-profile examples are Lynne Robinson, who was at the forefront of creating the Pilates boom in this country (and even taught the Chelsea football team), and Barbara Currie, a wonderful yoga teacher who at the age of seventy-four has been practising since she was twenty-nine and looks incredible for her age. You can find their details on page 232.

Back bends are Barbara's favourite 'anti-ageing' stretch as they improve posture, work out major muscles and improve that unflattering stoop that can develop in older age. For beginners, Barbara recommends the cobra pose: Lie on your stomach with your hands placed under your shoulders then press up slowly to arch your back. Keep the spine lengthened, shoulders down and focus on the back and front of the body.

STAY STRONG

Leading personal trainer Michael Garry says there are three simple stretches we should all do every single day as we get older to protect back, leg and hip mobility:

- Touch your toes with feet placed at shoulder width apart with a slight bend at the front of the knees. This will stretch hamstrings and help relieve any stress in the lower back region.

- Stretch your quads by standing on one leg (hold onto the back of a chair for balance if needed) and tuck your foot up by holding the front of your ankle and pulling it up behind you into your backside. Repeat on the other side.

- Stretch out your calves by standing on a step or on the bottom stair and letting the heels drop until you feel a deep stretch up through the calf muscles.

IN SUMMARY

- There are now plenty of minimally invasive cosmetic procedures which are not permanent but can give a much-needed boost to how we look and feel.

- There are also plenty of tricks to pick up on how to make ourselves look better – from using richer hand cream and addressing our posture to keeping ourselves flexible with daily stretches and bends.

- See the difference with my go-to skin regime for menopause skin.

CHAPTER SIX:
Sex (and Relationships)

Who doesn't want to be blessed with a wonderful relationship and to enjoy a life of healthy, fulfilling sex? For most of us, there will be, along the way, unsettling fluctuations in how we feel about ourselves and our partner, which may in turn affect the relationship negatively. During the menopause, these feelings may well be hormone-related – but not always – and I think it's important not to let ourselves believe (or be persuaded by others) that every decision we make at this stage of our lives is hormonally driven.

Our attitude towards sex may change for an exhaustive list of reasons, many psychological, many physiological, and be further complicated by our emotional reaction to these. It is also exceptionally hard to feel sexy, bold and excited about sex when you feel the opposite and may even feel reluctant to engage for fear of it hurting due to vaginal dryness causing friction and bleeding, or a little leak, a recurrence of thrush or (another) urinary tract infection.

These feelings are incredibly common and numerous experts in this field agree that our greatest challenge is to accept ourselves – that is, our *changing* selves – and to keep talking to our partner. I wanted to talk about all the things that might contribute to you not wanting sex or enjoying it – from increased flatulence to pelvic pain.

Of course, we all know exceptions among us – those who roar through the menopause with the libido of Catherine the Great, who never look invisible at parties and glow no matter how little sleep they get – but I don't really think they need any pointers (just our admiration!).

The sorry fact is that women's sexual functioning does decline with age but the science jury is still out as to whether this is actually due to the menopause, ageing, or other physical, psychological or social factors. Researchers from North Carolina found that women experienced a decline in libido twenty months before their last period and this was despite more than 75 per cent of them reporting that sex was moderately to extremely important to them. So, there is a disconnect between wanting sex, believing sex to be important, and actually having sex – but scientists have not decided why.

This study examined data on approximately 1,400 women and found that up until one year after their last period, sexual function fell 0.35 per cent and continued to decline for more than a year afterwards. And women who had a hysterectomy before the menopause didn't have a loss of libido before the procedure but did for as long as five years afterwards. [1]

What happened to my libido?

It's obvious to all of us now that when our hormone levels fall into decline it can have a significant impact on our desire for sex and that various physical changes may have an impact on how we feel about sex. This is especially true as our testosterone levels fall away.

With the reduction of collagen to keep the vagina elastic and flexible, it may shrink and expand less easily, making sex less spontaneous. The vulva (the external genitals – labia, clitoris and entrance to the vagina) may become thin, dry and itchy, and you may notice a reddening and soreness of the vulva or vagina, either occasionally or more often than not.

The pH balance of the vagina also changes. When younger and fertile, it is acidic to keep infections at bay in order to encourage conception. Now oestrogen is no longer dominant, there may be an increased risk of recurrent vaginal infections such as thrush, UTIs and itching. These problems are not reserved for those of us who are sexually active – it can happen to any of us.

More problems can occur if you have diabetes as the condition can damage the nerves of the cells lining the vagina, which in turn can interfere with arousal and orgasm, so if this does cause a problem then it is definitely time to see a specialist. If you find yourself with exceptionally dry skin, lethargy and weight gain then low libido may be a symptom of an underactive thyroid gland and it is a good idea to see your GP and get it checked out with a blood test.

Natural libido lifters

A healthy diet rich in Omega-3 and vitamin C may help boost the libido. If you take a multivitamin, make sure it includes zinc, which supports the sex hormones – French women swear by oysters as an aphrodisiac as they are packed with zinc. Vitamin C is key in collagen production, which softens both the skin on the face and the skin down below. The herb St John's wort is often taken for mild depression and some women say it helps their libido too. Taking testosterone is likely to make the most significant difference (see page 46).

Vaginal dryness

Another symptom of the menopause that I would suggest you may like to see your GP about it is vaginal dryness. So many women don't seek help because they are embarrassed, don't realise how common it is or feel they should just put up with it as there is nothing to be done. Treating vaginal dryness can bring a huge improvement to the quality of your life and that of your partner, so always make the time to seek advice from your GP.

While many of the problems surrounding sex at this age (UTIs, thrush, infections) are dealt with privately, with partners kept in the dark, vaginal dryness is so obvious to both parties it is not one you can hide from! If penetration is literally impossible and can't take place then it can lead to frustration and upset unless a solution is found.

Vaginal dryness, or atrophic vaginitis, is the result of a significant decrease in oestrogen levels. Oestrogen is responsible for keeping the vagina soft, flexible and lubricated – ready for sex and ready for conception. Some doctors refer to it as a genitourinary syndrome of menopause (GSM) because it's not just the vagina that is targeted – the urinary tract can also suffer.

This awful and common problem is thought to affect around 70 per cent of menopausal women, with symptoms such as itching, burning and discomfort. Although this is definitely exacerbated during sex, some women even find it uncomfortable carrying out everyday activities such as sitting down or walking. Vaginal dryness can also be caused by factors other than oestrogen levels, such as taking the pill, antidepressants, allergy and cold medications, as well as tamoxifen.

SOLUTIONS

1. Probiotics

- This is really when probiotics come into their own – not only for gut health but for good vaginal health. Taking a probiotic will increase the levels of good bacteria in the digestive system, which may help guard against thrush and vaginal and urinary infections, the plague of so many women during the menopause. The strains of L. rhamnosus and L. reuteri are believed to be especially effective here.

2. Lubrication

- If sex becomes really tricky because of vaginal dryness, do see your GP, who can prescribe a topical oestrogen either as a pessary, cream or vaginal ring. This takes a few weeks to work on softening the delicate vaginal tissue but it is effective. Be aware that it's completely safe to use vaginal oestrogen alongside HRT.

- If you prefer an OTC approach, always use a lube that's designed for the vagina – now is not the time to experiment with anything from the kitchen cupboard!

- Avoid anything too synthetic or too perfumed that may cause irritation, especially the stimulating varieties.

- The pH is important too; if it's too alkaline it can lead to UTIs or an occurrence of thrush, so check that it's between pH3.8 and pH4.5. Oil-based ones are not suitable with condoms but otherwise are fine. Most of us know of KY jelly, and it's what some doctors use for internal examinations, but it's not a great lube for vaginal dryness. YES is one that friends recommend, plus Replens, Sylk or Regelle. Don't be shy – this is also a great opportunity to discuss symptoms with your partner, who may be pleasantly surprised to find it enhances their own experiences.

3. Oestrogen

- Vaginal oestrogen is the most effective treatment here (this is different from HRT). In addition, taking HRT alone can usually make a huge difference to this symptom. About 20 per cent of women affected need systemic HRT as well as vaginal oestrogen – according to the menopause specialist Dr Louise Newson, having both together is very safe.

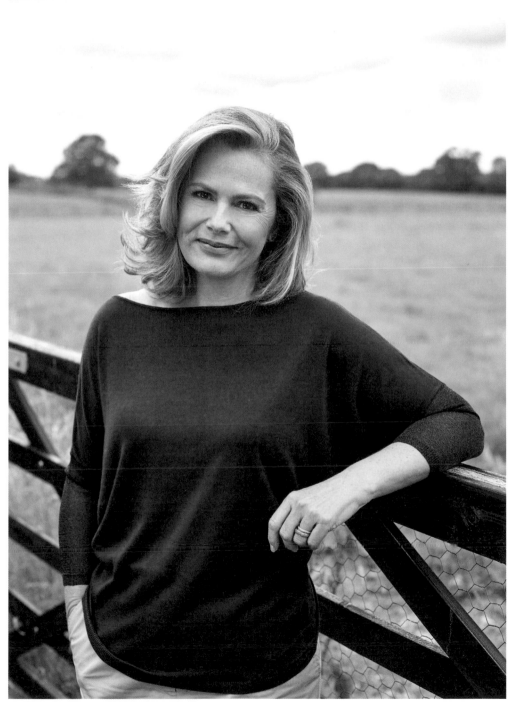

Ditch the itch

There can be few things more distressing than developing sensitivity around the vagina, but it does happen and it happens very often. Changes to the area can take months or even years to develop and, as skin becomes increasingly delicate, it is more likely to itch. And scratching an itch on your nose is one thing, but really? It is a truly awful symptom but there are measures you can take to lessen the itch as well as the risk of itch.

Always use gentle, non-scented soaps and pH-balanced washes for cleaning in this area, although you may find that water is all you need. Synthetic chemical products, including biological washing powder, bath and shower gels plus scented panty liners, may exacerbate the problem. Always wear cotton or natural-fibre underwear that fits well but isn't too tight (thong days may be gone!), and the same goes for tights and clothing, especially jeans.

If you find that thrush is a recurrent problem and the itching is exacerbated, then try eliminating sugar from your diet as this can trigger an overgrowth of yeast and contribute to feminine itching.

Flatulence

I'm afraid there's another delightful symptom of the menopause that needs to be tackled … Thanks to our hormones being in flux, we may produce more stomach gas – which means we may pass more wind. Worrying about it is not conducive to enjoying carefree sex, but there are a few solutions to try.

This process of excessive gas kicks off during the perimenopause, when the balance of good and bad bacteria involved in the digestive process is disrupted by the fluctuating levels of oestrogen and progesterone. When bacteria in the gut is balanced then healthy digestion occurs, but when patterns are altered the stomach reacts by increasing the production of gas. Obviously, the optimal solution is to balance hormone levels, but there are also other practical ways to help reduce stomach gas.

SOLUTIONS

- Eat smaller portions of food more frequently (eating large portions less often can lower digestive function).

- Chew food more slowly. This will break it down into smaller chunks and allow the digestive enzymes in saliva to work efficiently. Chew each mouthful twenty to thirty times before swallowing.

- Many of the fabulous foods I recommend for tackling other symptoms of the menopause – beans, lentils, wholewheat flour, etc – are great for gas! So, if this is a struggle, then do cut back on these foods to see if it makes a difference.

- Take a probiotic supplement to boost the levels of beneficial gut bacteria – which is helpful for all-round good health in any case. Choose a capsule or powder that contains several different strains of beneficial microflora with at least six to ten varieties.

- Exercise regularly. With the increased flow of blood through the body, the digestive system is stimulated to work more efficiently. This problem seems to affect the more sedentary among us, so being active will improve this symptom – and give you more confidence overall!

Quality not quantity

Many women feel sexually liberated after the menopause because they are no longer at risk of pregnancy, so find it an exciting time to explore the strong emotional bond that comes from sexual intimacy with their partner.

In her book, *Sex After Sixty*, author Marie de Hennezel explains how she feels women have a natural gift for erotic intimacy and also a responsibility to show their partner how much pleasure they take in being with them, and to help create a kind of erotic complicity that is both tender and gentle. As they get older, she says, men can become vulnerable and may be scared of losing their virility.

With this in mind I find the results of an American study heartening – and frankly hope the findings are true for all my friends. It discovered that although some women and their partners do report lower libidos after the menopause, they were experiencing the best sex of their lives.[2] They rated sexual satisfaction as higher at midlife, even if they had sex less often. Why? They said they had better knowledge and understanding of their bodies and how they work when it comes to sex, which in turn made them feel more comfortable and secure in their relationship.

Dr Anand Patel is a GP specialising in sexual problems in men and women of all ages and is extremely positive about sex for the older generations. His research shows that most women aged 50–59 are sexually active, with a fifth of all *octogenarians* enjoying some form of an active sex life. Dr Patel also explains how oestrogen can have a tremendous impact upon sexual touch, so our partner may notice that what once turned us on before the menopause is no longer invited or indeed may even be a turn-off. Thus, learning a new body landscape is key, although using HRT (plus or minus testosterone) can be hugely beneficial for some.

Too tired for sex?

Some of my friends swear by melatonin for insomnia and bring back supplies from trips to the US where they buy it OTC (and use for jetlag). Here it is available as a prescription-only medication for those who are fifty-five and over. It's a hormone synthesised by the pineal glands and has a critical role in the regulation of our circadian rhythms. It triggers chemical receptors in the brain to encourage sleep and limited research shows it may also help with short-term memory. A decent night's sleep is essential if we want to feel happy in ourselves, never mind amorous towards our partner.

Power up the pelvic floor

As we wave goodbye to the wonderful oestrogen, it's time to point out that it also had a role to play in keeping our bladder and urethra healthy. Our pelvic floor muscles surround the bladder and require oestrogen to keep it healthy and tight. As levels of the hormone fall, the pelvic floor slackens (which can be exacerbated if we are overweight) and this may allow bacteria to enter the bladder more freely, resulting in infection. Not to mention the range of bladder issues that can result from a weak pelvic floor, such as leaking when you sneeze, cough or laugh, urge incontinence and bladder irritation.

Stress urinary incontinence (SUI) is the most common type of incontinence but it is difficult to measure as many women never seek help. However, it is speculated that 50 per cent of forty-eight-year-olds experience it.[4] Yet the stronger our pelvic floor, the less likely we are to leak – plus we are more likely to enjoy a fulfilling sex life.

The series of exercises designed to work our pelvic floor – or Kegels – may have come in useful after childbirth to help prevent little leaks, but never have some of us wished we'd practised more than when we reached the menopause! One friend who had her babies by Caesarean, so hadn't pushed them through the birth canal, didn't think she needed to work on her pelvic floor and now says she frantically uses every water-cooler moment in the office to lift and squeeze.

The pelvic floor is a sheet of muscles that extends from our tail bone, or coccyx, to our pubic bone at the front, forming a platform between our legs. It provides the floor to our pelvis and the lower portion of our tummy, and supports the contents of our pelvis – the bladder, uterus and back passage. It also controls the openings of the following organs which pass through it: the urethra – the tube through which urine is delivered – the vagina and birth canal, and the anus, through which we open our bowels.

Signs of a weakened pelvic floor include an aching or dragging sensation in the vagina, a feeling of something coming down inside the vagina, and a tendency to leak when you cough, laugh or sneeze (SUI). You may suffer from frequency to urinate during the day or night and urge incontinence, when you need to visit the loo but leak before you get there.

What can make the pelvic floor weak? There's quite a list so here goes: childbirth, a lack of exercise, the menopause, a hysterectomy, bladder repair, straining to open your bowels, being overweight.

Pelvic floor exercises will help strengthen the muscles so that they can give our organs support again. This will improve bladder control and improve or stop any leakage.

1. Close and draw up the muscles around your anus as if trying to stop passing wind, but do not contract buttock muscles while doing so.

2. Now close and draw up the muscles around your vagina and urethra, as though trying to stop the flow of urine. Hold for as long as possible, then slowly relax and let go.

3. Slowly increase the length of time that you hold each contraction for and do as many as you can until you feel the muscle getting tired.

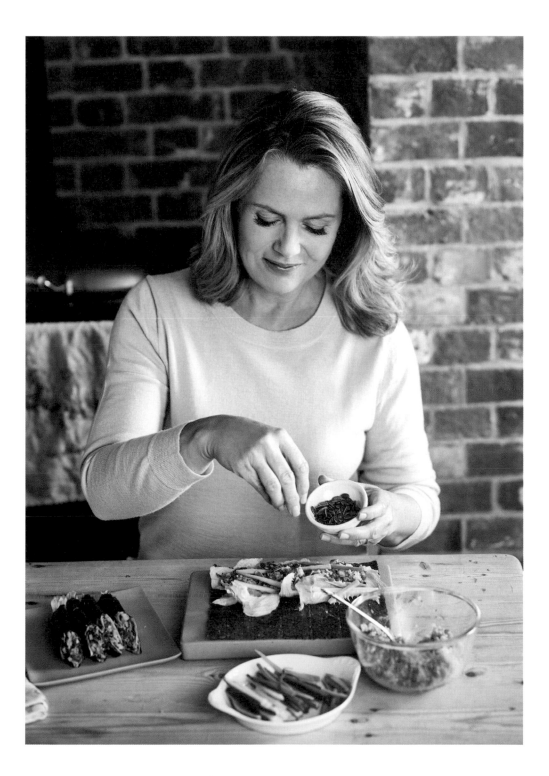

You should ideally aim to do your pelvic floor exercises on a daily basis, and fewer good squeezes are better than lots of mediocre ones. You can also test your pelvic floor muscles during sex by squeezing hard and seeing how long you can hold it for – and gradually extend the length with practice.

And finally, always try to brace the pelvic floor muscles by squeezing up and holding your pelvic floor contraction before you cough, laugh, sneeze, lift anything heavy, or prior to any activity that may make you leak. Be patient as it will take weeks of exercise to supersize your pelvic floor muscles, but you must keep working them *forever* otherwise problems will return.

Pelvic pain

Given that our reproductive system is effectively retiring, we might be forgiven for thinking that our days of tummy ache and stabbing pains and bloating would be over. Wrong! Chronic pelvic pain can truly disrupt some women's lives and is caused by any number of gynaecological problems, such as benign or malignant tumours, pelvic adhesions or interstitial cystitis. However, the most common cause of pelvic pain among postmenopausal women is fibroids.

Fibroids are benign pelvic tumours and tend to be slow-growing, so it can take months or even years for them to cause any problems. Although many are asymptomatic and cause little or no pain or bleeding, some can trigger abnormal uterine bleeding, pelvic pain, constipation, back pain, pressure on the bladder and fertility problems. Fibroids are responsible for nearly a third of hysterectomies each year.

Fibroids contain both oestrogen and progesterone receptors and respond to any type of hormonal stimulation so may grow when hormones fluctuate, such as during the menopause. While the menopause can in some cases see fibroids shrinking, they can also begin to cause even more pelvic pain, particularly in those who take HRT as the hormones can sometimes stimulate fibroid growth.

IN SUMMARY

- Focus on quality of sex not quantity – studies have shown we CAN enjoy a fulfilled love life into old age.

- Take probiotics for good gut health – and to combat flatulence as the stomach may now produce more gas.

- Power up the pelvic floor – every day! This will give you more confidence during sex and help with any little leaks.

CHAPTER SEVEN:
Emotions

Our emotional landscape can become difficult to navigate during the perimenopause and menopause. Suddenly the changes in our body lead us to question who we are, what our role is in life, and ask where on earth are we going and with whom. The confidence we built up in our twenties and thirties seems shaken and we may start to feel anxious about seemingly trivial things and begin to worry.

We may not feel like ourselves, and spend a tremendous amount of time thinking of how we might get back to 'being me'. Yet as most doctors will tell us, the menopause is simply another milestone, so perhaps we ought to rail against it less, despite wanting to fight it all the way. But as natural as this stage of our lives may be, I have yet to meet anyone who says it *feels* natural; rather they describe it as like having a rug suddenly pulled from under them (although one friend says it was like a rug being thrown over them!).

Successful women I know who are physically and emotionally resilient feel robbed of their usual drive and determination, doubting themselves and lacking in confidence. Others have been crippled by mood swings which have affected the whole family, endured hot flushes which have left them not wanting to socialise and ended up with a crushed libido which they can't (and often don't want to) revive.

The psychological symptoms attached to the menopause, such as low self-esteem, anxiety and irritability, are every bit as gruelling as the physical symptoms. Inextricably linked, they can have a domino effect not only on the body but on relationships, at home and work. So, for example, insomnia can lead to a foggy head the next day, a feeling of irritability and an exhaustion that means you don't feel quite right and are more likely to burst into tears or lose your temper over something trivial. Overtired, you may crave salt, sugar or caffeine, not to mention the odd glass of wine to prop you up, leading to weight gain, bloating and a despair that your body is generally conspiring against you.

You may find that your mood takes a real dive so that you end up feeling low more often than not – a sort of bleak, ongoing PMS – and it's incredibly helpful to realise that this is a very, very common symptom during the perimenopause and menopause, yet is not the same as having clinical depression. However, if postnatal depression has been diagnosed in the past, then it's as well to be aware that your symptoms could be extreme during the menopause as the body becomes more sensitive to changing levels of hormones.

Hormonal changes and antidepressants

By now you may be forgiven for thinking that oestrogen is the elixir of life and can cure anything – well, it is pretty powerful stuff – but it does not treat clinical depression, although it can help it. One study of depressed elderly women showed greater improvement in the group treated with oestrogen and fluoxetine (selective serotonin reuptake inhibitor – SSRI) than in those treated with oestrogen alone or a placebo, suggesting that oestrogen may increase the antidepressant effect.[1]

However, many women find themselves wrongly prescribed antidepressants by their GP for symptoms which, although similar to those of depression, are common with the menopause, which further highlights how little awareness there is even among doctors. Medication for a mood disorder won't be able to deal with mood-related symptoms that are due to hormonal changes. A report from NHS Digital in June 2017 found that there has been a 108 per cent rise in prescriptions for antidepressants in the past ten years, to 64.7 million, and that GPs are handing out the drugs too readily, with more than 1 million patients in the UK taking them needlessly. Interestingly, this timeline coincides with the era when so many middle-aged women were advised to stop taking HRT due to the wrongly reported breast cancer scare studies.

Although research shows some success in antidepressants treating vasomotor symptoms such as hot flushes, more work needs to be carried out. Common side effects of SSRIs include feeling agitated, shaky or anxious, dizziness, insomnia, headaches and low libido. HRT can improve some of the low feelings related to menopause and many of the other psychological symptoms such as irritability, low self-esteem and anxiety. How many, I wonder, of the patients taking antidepressants are actually menopausal and could so easily benefit from topping up their dwindling hormones by taking HRT instead?

Why CBT therapy works

For all those keen to treat symptoms without medication it is as well to know that current NICE guidelines recommend cognitive behavioural therapy (CBT), and leading therapist Anna Albright explains why it is an effective alternative during such a stressful phase.

'We experience physiological changes and psychological changes in the menopause and CBT deals with the emotional changes as a result of those. I may see women who, for example, have empty-nest syndrome or loss of libido and there is a grieving process which takes time as they reconcile themselves to change. Once we are conscious of the problems then we can develop a healthy response to them.

'We all trade on some "thing" – it might be our brain, our personality, figure or our face. When that "thing" goes as it inevitably does, we have to come to terms with the fact it's only going one way. It opens up a bigger existential question – who or what are we when that "thing", which is most often our looks, goes?

'We need to come to the realisation that there is no quick fix. It's not a broken leg and we can't see it or touch it or mend it. We have scant understanding of this phase in our lives and the adjustment from perimenopause, through menopause to post menopause goes on for many years as our entire chemistry and function changes and this process takes a few years to come to terms with. CBT explores these changes and works on coping strategies and a way through these changes.'

Be positive!

So, how much of our experience of the menopause is down to our personality? Scientists say we *can* do a tremendous amount to help ourselves, according to a review of studies, which concluded that if we have a more positive attitude towards the menopause then we will actually suffer less. Researchers found that in ten out of thirteen studies, women who held negative attitudes towards the menopause also reported having more problems with menopausal symptoms.[2]

Feelings of inadequacy and self-criticism also appear to escalate during the menopause. In a review of more than thirty studies, Joan C. Chrisler, Professor of Psychology at Connecticut College, and Varda Muhlbauer of Netanya Academic College in Israel noticed a curious link between negativity and appearance. When women were asked to rate how they felt about their bodies, menopausal women tended to judge themselves negatively, yet when asked general questions about their lives, these same women reported a high level of satisfaction. So, 'life is good but what happened to my body and my brain?' seems to be the general consensus.[3]

I am aware that studies such as these tend to lump us all together, yet each of us will experience the menopause differently and it's so important not to make comparisons with others going through it. We should support one another in finding a way through.

Facing up to fear and anger

It may feel daunting to seek professional help for the menopause together with your partner, but sex counsellors at Relate, the UK's largest provider of relationship support, are experienced in helping couples understand that the menopause is a natural and normal milestone in a woman's life. They cite fear and anger as two of the key emotions that may be felt by both partners.

Other factors that may be adding stress include empty-nest feelings, retirement, poor health and looking after elderly parents. Relate's advice is to reassess the partnership: as energy levels and motivations change, couples may need to discuss their roles in the household and who does what, especially if depression becomes an issue.

Relate recommends we listen to concerns, fears and frustrations and be there for our partner. They urge us to be patient, with our partner and ourselves, if mood swings occur or if forgetfulness is an issue. We know that exercise may help reduce some menopausal symptoms but Relate emphasises the 'together' aspect of managing change, so joining an exercise class *together*, going for a swim or walk *together*, is well worth trying. The real emphasis here is on all concerns and changes – and that it's not just the woman who's changing at this time of life.

The male menopause

This is probably a good moment to touch on our menfolk and whether or not the time of life they are going through affects them in any parallel way. The 'male menopause' is also called andropause and is a time when men experience a drop in their testosterone levels. This can cause many symptoms, including depression or low mood, a loss of self-confidence, hair loss, insomnia, reduced muscle mass, increased 'middle-aged spread' or a paunch, and erectile dysfunction.

The options for guys here are similar to ours in many ways – they should always discuss symptoms with their doctor (although relatively few actually do) and they may be prescribed counselling, hormone replacement therapy (in the form of testosterone) or possibly antidepressants. It's no wonder that when two people in a relationship are going through such a similar time their relationship can so easily suffer as a result.

Feel better at work

It's all well and good taking care of ourselves at home but most women will find themselves working through the menopause. They've been a long time coming but new practical guidelines were finally introduced in 2016 to help support women and their colleagues and managers in tackling the occupational aspects of menopausal symptoms.[4]

The guidelines are based on those produced by the European Menopause and Andropause Society (EMAS) and include workplace training to increase awareness of the potential effects of menopause, adapting the workplace environment where appropriate (for example, changing the temperature of offices and having fans available), making flexible hours for some women an option and, perhaps most importantly, creating opportunities to facilitate discussion about symptoms that are impacting on the ability to work.

Clear guidance is also given for women themselves, which includes encouraging discussions to take place with managers and the occupational health service about practical needs plus talking to colleagues. It is also recommended that women do not suffer in silence and that they seek advice regarding available treatment, such as HRT, from their GP.

Hair loss and self-esteem

I wanted to talk about hair here (see also the chapter on beauty) because it is such an emotive issue for all women going through the menopause. Our relationship with hair is complex and primal. An abundance of healthy, shiny locks is a wonderful reflection of youth and fertility, while menopause and thinning hair are often associated with loss of femininity and sexuality and, sadly, to a certain extent this is true.

Please remember that although at times it may feel as if you are losing your crowning glory, it's very rare to go bald and it is considered normal to lose 100 hairs a day whatever our age. Androgenetic alopecia may see hair thinning on top and at the temples, where a loss of oestrogen causes androgens – the male hormones – to become more dominant. And this gives us another reason to have a magnifying mirror – facial hair!

The upset caused by thinning, barely there hair for all the world to see may contribute to hair loss, as may being deficient in certain nutrients such as iron. Hair is mainly made up of protein and we need to consume it in plentiful amounts plus ensure we are on top of our B-complex vitamins and biotin (found in egg yolks, lentils, brown rice, soya beans and sunflower seeds). If hair loss is severely affecting your social life, your mood and your behaviour changes as a result, then it is time to talk to your GP about a referral to a trichologist and discuss options for treatment.

Don't let memory loss kill confidence

I am not alone when I say confidence can really take a knocking if you feel muddle-headed and your memory seems worryingly bad. Why is it that forgetfulness is such an issue during the menopause? Oestrogen regulates levels of the hormone cortisol, which in turn affects brain chemicals, so as oestrogen levels dip the control it has over cortisol can be erratic, resulting in short-term memory lapses.

It's common not to feel (or want to be) as engaged as once before; overcome by a sense of ennui, the ability to concentrate or multitask also wanes. You may find yourself asking: Am I becoming lazier? Is this what old age is going to be like? Do I have early-onset dementia? It's reassuring to remember that these are very common symptoms, and many are the stories of doing ridiculously silly things like putting dishwasher tablets in the washing machine, trying to cancel a bank card already cancelled the day before and forgetting where we parked the car twenty minutes earlier (we walked).

While we know that falling hormone levels can contribute to these symptoms, it's also important to acknowledge and give ourselves credit for dealing with these seismic changes at what is an incredibly busy time of life for many of us: having a responsible job, caring and/or parenting commitments and possibly volunteering and community projects. Don't be too self-critical – and do keep talking to family and friends.

Plan the perfect time to eat

It makes complete sense that we should all eat breakfast to keep blood sugar levels steady and eat protein to ensure we don't have a slump after eating simple carbohydrates such as toast or pastries. Boiled or poached eggs with avocado, yoghurt and/or kefir are my own personal favourites. That said, carbohydrates are thought to increase the amount of serotonin in the brain, which has a calming effect, but choose food with complex carbohydrates, such as wholegrains like quinoa, wholegrain breads and wholegrain cereals.

Sleep expert Dr Nerina Ramlakhan explains in her book *Fast Asleep, Wide Awake* that sleep problems aren't created when we put our head on the pillow but that everything we do during the day, and every choice we make, can have an impact on how we sleep at night. One of her non-negotiables is eating breakfast within thirty to forty-five minutes of getting up as it stabilises blood sugar, and she says we won't then need to rely on stress hormones to keep us going. Plus we will start to make more of the sleep hormone melatonin and, in doing so, she says, sleep better.

Observe regular mealtimes and plan menus with fresh fruit and fresh vegetables – and don't overeat. Dehydration is often overlooked, so aim to keep topped up with plenty of water all day. Tea and coffee can make us feel wonderful momentarily, only to leave us jittery and sapping the body of energy. Their diuretic properties can also rob the body of much-needed minerals, such as calcium. Stick to one or two cups in the morning as a maximum.

One other reason not to overdo refined carbohydrates is shown in a study by the department of psychiatry at the University of Columbia, which concluded that a diet rich in high-glycaemic foods, such as processed white breads, biscuits, cereals and white rice, may lead to a greater risk of first-onset depression in postmenopausal women.[5] So try to stick to a low GI diet (with the recipes in this book) pretty much all of the time.

Boost your mood with serotonin – the happy neurotransmitter

Serotonin is found in blood platelets and serum and is a neurotransmitter that can affect appetite, mood, digestion, sleep, memory and libido. It was only relatively recently discovered that 90 per cent of our serotonin lives in the gut and is produced when we eat protein-rich foods containing the amino acid tryptophan. Spinach and watercress are rich in tryptophan – far more so than turkey, duck, quail or pork – although the best source of all is spirulina, the blue-green algae which can be added to juices and smoothies. Tryptophan converts to a substance called 5-HTP in the brain and can be bought as a supplement to help ease low moods.

WALNUTS

Nuts are excellent sources of protein and healthy fats, and one type of nut in particular might also improve memory. A 2015 study from UCLA linked higher walnut consumption to improved cognitive test scores. Walnuts are high in a type of Omega-3 fatty acid called alpha-linolenic acid (ALA), which helps lower blood pressure and protects arteries.

Yoga – what's not to like?

One inspiring champion of the menopause in the US is Sara Gottfried, a gynaecologist who teaches natural hormone balancing and author of *The Hormone Cure* and *The Hormone Reset Diet*. She's also a qualified yoga teacher.

Not only does yoga decrease cortisol and adrenaline (the main stress hormones), Sara says she noticed that it reduced the fat on her tummy (and she was nicer to her husband). We have, she says, four times more receptors for cortisol stored in our tummy fat, than elsewhere on the body. She also explains that yoga raises melatonin levels after three months of practice, which may help with restorative sleep and also correct the thyroid, prolactin, luteinising and follicle-stimulating hormones. And how long before you can expect to see a difference? Practise for five days a week for thirty to sixty minutes and after between three and six months you should be feeling more lean and serene. Worth a go I think – and there are plenty of apps and online tutorials if you can't get to a regular class nearby.

Oh oxytocin!

Of all the wonderful hormones that surge during motherhood, oxytocin – or the love hormone, as it's also called – is the most powerful. It is a neurotransmitter and is stimulated during sex, childbirth and breastfeeding and helps release feelings of empathy and generosity. What a shame then that this caring, sharing, touchy-feely hormone also dwindles with the menopause. On some basic level, it makes sense – we no longer need to reproduce or breastfeed or rear children, so those maternal instincts can take a back seat.

Perhaps this is why during the menopause years some women decide to take their lives in a completely different direction and go for the ultimate in 'me-time' – 66 per cent of divorces that occur between the ages of forty and sixty-nine are initiated by women. In her book *The Female Brain*, neuropsychiatrist Dr Louann Brizendine explains that when we are menopausal we are less bothered about keeping the peace and less inclined to be as attentive to others' needs and, rather, we become more attuned to our own desires. Interesting new studies are now linking the beneficial bacteria strain *L. reutari* with boosted oxytocin production.

Make mine a massage

Can we recreate that loving hormone, though? One small study from UCLA showed that massage does increase a release of oxytocin and concluded that although it is still not understood fully how, social interaction and touch have an impact on stress hormones and morbidity.[6]

Another study measured the effect of a scalp massage for stress therapy. A scalp massage was given to 34 female office workers twice a week for 10 weeks on stress hormones, blood pressure and heart rate in healthy women. Significant differences were recorded in norepinephrine, cortisol and blood pressure and researchers concluded that scalp massage can be used positively for stress control.[7]

If you haven't given massage a go before, you may feel quite self-conscious even trying it out on a partner, but perhaps the secret is to start on yourself, maybe on your head and feet and then on your partner. If you'd like to practise something that's more formal than instinctive, there are plenty of instructive tutorials and how-to video guides online.

And finally, I wish all of us the calm poise that Hollywood actress Angelina Jolie displayed when she wrote in the *New York Times* about her experience of the menopause, aged just thirty-nine, after her decision to have a double mastectomy plus her ovaries and fallopian tubes removed due to a family history of the BRCA genes and losing her mother to cancer:

'I am now in menopause. I will not be able to have any more children and I expect some physical changes. But I feel at ease with whatever will come, not because I am strong but because this is part of life. It is nothing to be feared.'

IN SUMMARY

- Take a look at how cognitive behavioural therapy can help with coming to terms with the menopause.

- Science has shown that a positive attitude can make all the difference to how we experience the menopause.

- Touch and massage can have an incredibly effect on lowering levels of stress and blood pressure so give it a go!

CHAPTER EIGHT:
Conclusions

If there is one thing I want you to take away from this book, other than a greater understanding and awareness of such a transformative phase in our lives, it is for you to be so much kinder to yourself.

We now live longer than any other previous generations and, for the most part, in better health, yet our lives are incredibly complicated as a result. We may be working while still raising a family and/or caring for elderly parents, and perhaps divorced or on a second or third marriage with stepchildren. To then introduce (and not at a time of our choosing) the tremendous physical and psychological changes which rampage through us at the menopause is a challenge that would floor most superheroes.

We need to give ourselves far more credit for simply keeping it all together and, when we can't, to put up our hand and ask for help. If the stigma of mental health issues can be overcome to make top billing across the media, government and the public, then so should the menopause!

Yet that can only happen if we also support and care for one another. We need to choose to talk more and to share both our wisdom and solutions. One of my friends says she felt the menopause was like childbirth – no one really tells you how bad it is and she regrets not asking her mother and friends for their advice and help.

As we confront the menopause head-on, we mustn't judge one another on the choices we make in order to face the future with confidence. Does it really matter if we choose to have a full facelift if it makes us feel better? Or perhaps we decide it's the perfect time for liposuction or to reduce or boost the size of our breasts? At a time when we may feel our bodies are falling apart or at least conspiring against us, is it any wonder we want to try to look our best? It's not that we want to look *different* or younger; we just want to stay the same.

The menopause is not only a family issue – it's a national issue (and global too, but small steps!). I do believe society is starting to wake up to the fact that, if we truly care for our older female population, then not only will our family life continue to flourish, we will have a healthy older female workforce, which in the long term helps reduce the burden on the NHS.

A brilliant example of how the workplace might adapt – comes from GP and menopause medical specialist Dr Louise Newson. She offers workshops to the older female police workforce across several counties, and devises strategies for and raises awareness of how the menopause might affect them.

How enlightened is that? Her findings report that 81 per cent of women said the menopause was affecting their ability at work and 10 per cent of women actually stop work because of their menopausal symptoms. Many organisations do now offer health and wellbeing strategies in the workplace to prevent staff sickness, boost morale and enhance performance, so it would make so much sense to include training not only around pregnancy, mental health issues and disability, but also the menopause.

However, we still don't have a driving force within the NHS of GPs who have the right training or feel confident in treating patients suffering from the menopause. This means anyone turning up at their surgery with menopausal symptoms similar to anxiety and depression, which are common problems dealt with by GPs, might be offered antidepressants in the first instance – which may help some women but they do not actually address the physical menopausal problem.

In London, there are NHS menopause clinics at Queen Charlotte's and Chelsea Hospital, part of the Imperial College NHS Healthcare Trust, which offer care for women with routine and complex menopause-related gynaecological, medical and hormonal therapy problems. There are other dedicated NHS menopause clinics across the country, but waiting lists are long.

The NHS released new figures on obesity in June 2017 which really do make me fearful for the health of future generations. Four in ten young adults in Britain are overweight or obese – that's 3 million or 39 per cent of sixteen to twenty-four-year-olds who are putting their health at risk, a million more than twenty years ago. They risk dying at a younger age than us despite ongoing medical breakthroughs.

I worry for these overweight young women. Not only are they more likely to encounter fertility issues, as well as weight-related risks attached to pregnancy and birth, but when it then comes to the menopause, unless they have a normal BMI, they are likely to face further health problems such as diabetes, cancer and heart disease, never mind struggling to shift excess weight. When 23 per cent of these young women have a waist of 34.5 inches or more, then we are failing our children very badly indeed.

That's why we must take a positive stand and talk to our daughters more and encourage them to follow a healthier path – for their long-term health and happiness. And last, but not least, we need to stand alongside our sisterhood in sharing our own highs and lows, to bring menopause out of the mysterious darkness and into the bright shining light.

There are resources at the back of this book so please do join in, tell your friends and let's start a menopause movement – there's certainly enough of us to get involved!

PART TWO: RECIPES

Eating for Wellbeing

Food has such tremendous power to help and heal our changing bodies, especially in later life when we rely on greater levels of nutrition to sustain us as we age. The recipes that follow include plenty of especially helpful ingredients to create not only deliciously tasty, but also fantastically nourishing meals. All good for mid-life wellbeing, but which can also be enjoyed by everyone at any stage of life.

My special ingredients include phyto-oestrogens, which provide oestrogen-like compounds that occur naturally in the plant kingdom, to help ease many menopausal symptoms, but are also tasty and nutritious in their own right. Phyto-oestrogens include linseeds (also a good vegetarian source of Omega-3 essential fatty acids, vital for skin and brain health) and soya. I like using soya beans as a protein-rich vegetable (try mixing with peas as a side dish) as they also deliver a strong umami flavour that enhances other foods on the plate, as well as providing plenty of energy-boosting iron (especially when they're fermented soya beans). I've also shared some of my kitchen cupboard secrets, including cinnamon to help curb sugar cravings and even-out those mid-afternoon energy slumps. I use spelt as a more nutritious and more easily-digested grain; the spice turmeric for its anti-inflammatory properties as well as garlic for its anti-bacterial and general all-round health giving properties. Following on from the success of my previous book, *The Good Gut Guide*, I've added extra helpings of beneficial gut bacteria-boosting probiotics from plain, live yoghurt (also an excellent calcium-rich bone maintainer).

The recipe section starts with some great breakfast dishes to set us up for the day, as well as fabulous weekend brunch treats to share with family and friends. You'll find some lovely lunch and supper ideas, with plenty of veggie options (even a few vegan favourites of mine too) and everything can be easily adapted to be meat-free should you choose. I find that eating little and often can help boost flagging energy levels, so I've added some great snack ideas. Everything is designed to be relatively low GI (glycaemic index) to help maintain a steady energy balance throughout the day. And, of course, I've added a few sweet treats, free from refined sugars for something a little extra special too. I hope you love them all.

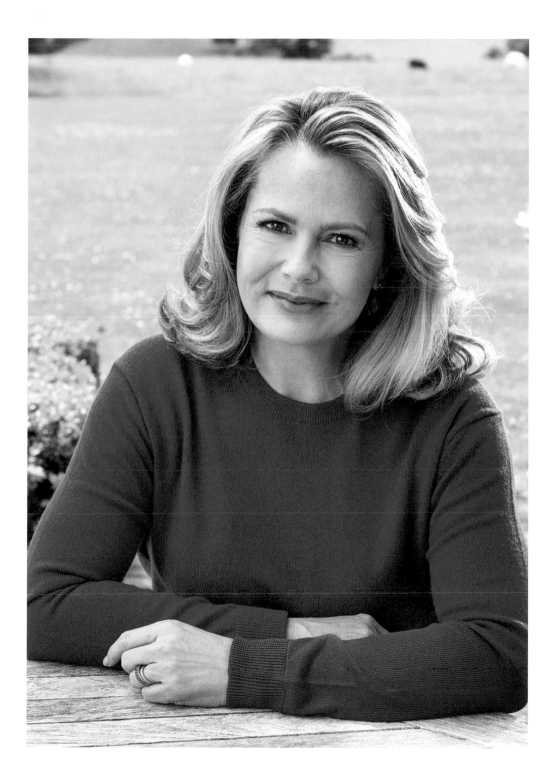

BREAKFAST

Summer berry pancakes

My healthy take on American pancakes are a big hit for weekend brunches or an indulgent summer dessert. Do try spelt flour – it's a good source of fibre, magnesium and iron and slightly easier to digest than wheat. Berries are a sweet source of antioxidants, while the dash of cinnamon may help curb sugar cravings.

(V) SERVES 2　　　　　　　　　　　　　　　　　　　　　　　　　　　　　329 calories

80g spelt flour

½ tsp baking powder

1 tsp ground cinnamon, plus extra to sprinkle

1 medium egg

75g plain live yoghurt, plus a little extra to serve

4–5 tbsp milk

150g summer berries (just thawed if using frozen)

15g butter

Drizzle of raw runny honey

- Sift the spelt into a bowl with the baking powder and cinnamon. Make a well in the middle and stir in the egg, yoghurt and milk. Carefully fold in the berries. Set aside for 10 minutes.

- Heat the butter in a large frying pan and spoon four spoonfuls of the mixture onto the pan – you should use all of it up. Cook over a low to medium heat for 2–3 minutes until the base has set, then flip over each pancake and cook the other side until the middle has set, too.

- Serve each pancake with a dollop of yoghurt, drizzle over a little honey and sprinkle with cinnamon.

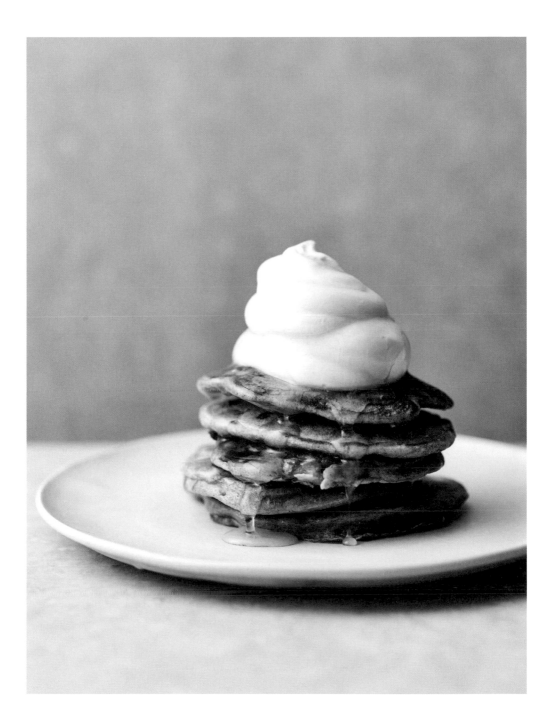

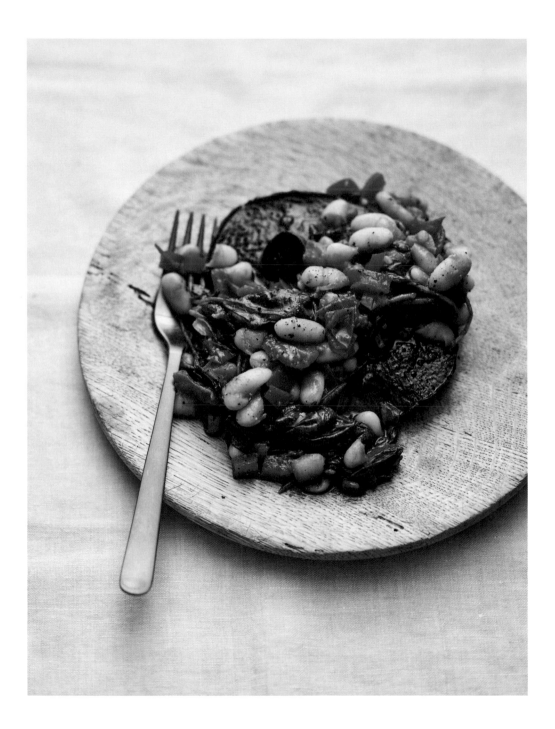

Veggie beans on grilled mushrooms

This works wonders as a weekend brunch dish – and the cooking aroma is incredible! I leave mushrooms on a windowsill to ripen for an hour, as this adds significant vitamin D. Cannellini beans are used in canned baked beans and are a great source of protein and fibre, but here they are without sugar and additives. Never miss a trick to boost metabolism by adding cayenne pepper or cinnamon, which may help curb sugar cravings.

V DF GF SERVES 2   163 calories

2 tsp olive oil
2 spring onions, finely chopped
10 cherry tomatoes, quartered
½ red pepper, deseeded and chopped
Good pinch ground cinnamon (or more to taste)
Good pinch cayenne pepper (or more to taste)

Sea salt and freshly ground black pepper
½ x 400g can cannellini beans, drained
1 tbsp tomato purée
4 large portobello/field mushrooms
1 tsp fresh or dried thyme
100g baby spinach leaves

- Preheat the grill.

- Heat half the oil in a pan and sauté the spring onions, tomatoes and red pepper for 5 minutes until softened, tossing the pan every now and then.

- Stir in the cinnamon and cayenne and season well. Cook for 1 minute. Stir in the beans, tomato purée and 75ml water. Cover and simmer over a low heat for 5 minutes.

- Put the mushrooms on a baking sheet with the stalks sitting up. Mix together the remaining oil and thyme and season well. Brush all over the mushrooms and grill for 5 minutes. Turn off the grill.

- Stir the spinach into the pan with the beans and cook until just wilted.

- Divide the mushrooms between two plates, spoon the beans evenly over the top and serve.

LIZ'S TIP

If you prefer, you can replace the cannellini beans with kidney beans.

Baked eggs

Eggs are one of the most nutrient-dense foods and, for an alternative to poached or boiled eggs, try this tasty dish. Besides being rich in vitamin D, riboflavin, vitamin B12 and iron, eggs are packed with protein. Let mushrooms ripen on a windowsill for an hour to boost the vitamin D in their skins. Using cooked tomatoes provides more lycopene than raw ones, as well as vitamin C, making this a powerful breakfast or light lunch.

(V) (DF) GF **SERVES 2**   248 calories

4 large portobello mushrooms

2 plum tomatoes, halved

1 tbsp olive oil

1 tsp fresh thyme leaves

Sea salt and freshly ground black pepper

4 medium eggs

- Preheat the oven to 190°C/375°F/Gas Mark 5.

- Arrange the mushrooms and tomatoes in a roasting tin, leaving space to crack in the eggs. You can snap off the mushroom stalks if you like and pop them in the tin as well. Mix the oil and thyme together and drizzle over the top. Season well.

- Bake in the oven for 10 minutes.

- Carefully crack the eggs into the tin. Bake for 6–8 minutes until set then serve.

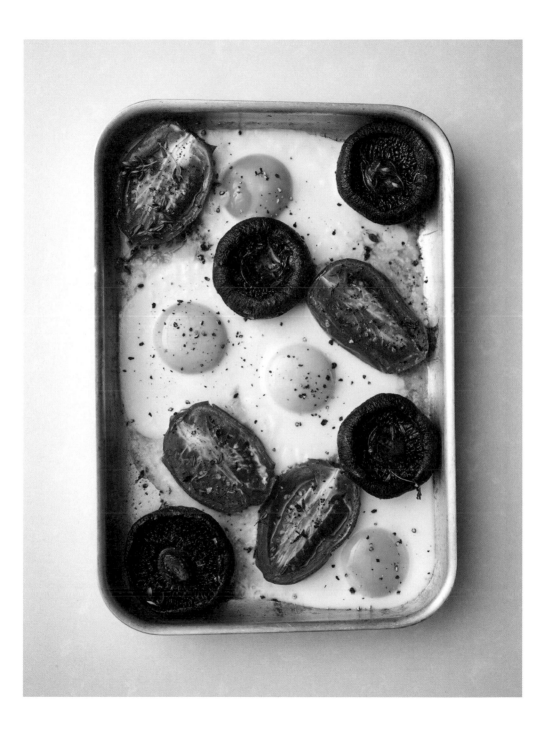

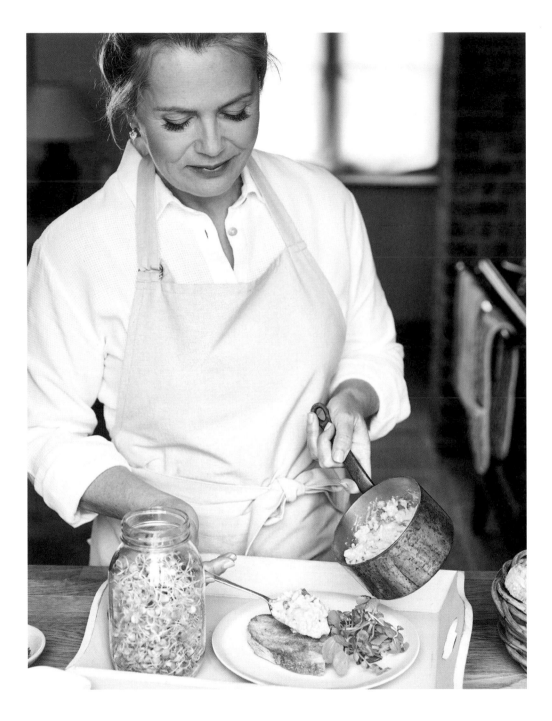

Scrambled eggs with sprouting lentils and watercress

For a delicious take on scrambled eggs – which are, of course, packed with protein, chromium and iron – add sprouting lentils for a colourful source of vitamin B, plus the sprouting actually produces vitamin C. Watercress adds a wonderful strong flavour and again adds iron, as well as the potential anti-cancer compound sulforaphane. This makes an ideal light lunch – even lighter without the sourdough bread.

Ⓥ SERVES 2   364 calories

75g sprouting lentils or seeds
40g watercress, chopped
Sea salt and freshly ground black pepper
Lemon wedge

Small knob of butter
4 medium eggs
2 slices sourdough bread or seeded loaf
  (page 205)

- Spoon the sprouting lentils or seeds into a bowl and add half the watercress. Season well and squeeze over the lemon. Toss to mix everything together then divide between two plates.

- Melt the butter in a pan over a medium heat and stir in the eggs. Continue to stir over a low to medium heat until the eggs have started to cook but are still a little bit runny. Add the remaining watercress then stir again and cook until creamy or until set the way you like them.

- While the eggs are cooking, toast the bread, if you like. Add a slice to each of the plates, spoon over the scrambled eggs and serve.

LIZ'S TIP

If you want to sprout your own lentils or seeds, here's how to do it. Measure 100g lentils into a bowl and pick out any bits – sometimes there's the odd stone in there. Wash well. Put in a large jar and cover with 300–400ml cold water – the jar should be around three-quarters full. Cover with muslin and secure with an elastic band or string tied round the neck of the jar. Leave to soak overnight. The next day, drain the water. Lay the jar on its side so it's horizontal on a kitchen draining board so any more liquid can drain away. Leave overnight. The next day, rinse again, and do this two to three times a day until the lentils start to sprout. This should happen in around 3 days.

Avocado, bean and ricotta smash on sourdough

This breakfast favourite is simple to make and, as sourdough is easy to digest, it won't make you feel sluggish. Avocado is packed with good fats, magnesium and B vitamins, ricotta provides protein, while the beans add fibre and will help you feel fuller for longer. As well as adding much-needed spice, cayenne pepper is a metabolism booster and turmeric is a powerful anti-inflammatory.

(V) GF SERVES 2   332 calories

½ large avocado

¼ tsp turmeric

Good pinch cayenne pepper

Juice of ½ lemon

100g canned cannellini beans, drained

75g ricotta or cottage cheese

Sea salt and freshly ground black pepper

2 slices good sourdough bread

½ tomato, finely chopped

A little freshly chopped parsley

1 tsp extra virgin olive oil

- Scrape the avocado flesh into a bowl and add the turmeric, cayenne and lemon juice. Mash well with the back of a fork until the avocado is almost smooth, with a few chunks left in it.

- Fold in the beans and ricotta or cottage cheese and season well.

- Spread the mixture over the slices of sourdough, then top each with half of the chopped tomato and parsley.

- Drizzle with the oil and finish with a little black pepper.

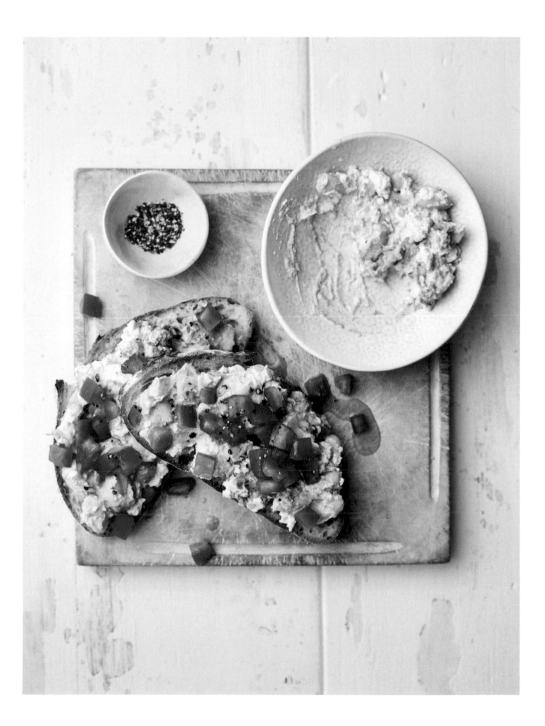

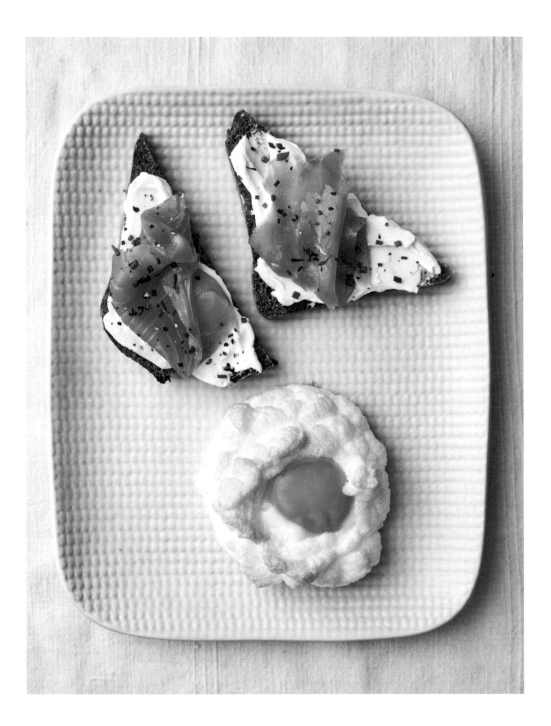

Smoked salmon on rye with cloud eggs

I save this pretty-as-a-picture egg dish for lunches with girlfriends or for a special brunch. While you don't need a large plate, the flavours stack up nicely, with salmon offering skin-saving protein, B vitamins, vitamin D and magnesium, and the eggs providing biotin.

SERVES 2   285 calories

2 large eggs
Pinch sea salt
2 tbsp freshly chopped chives
2 tbsp cream cheese

2 small slices dark rye bread
100g smoked salmon (preferably wild, not farmed, to avoid traces of anti-lice chemicals)
Freshly ground black pepper

- Preheat the oven to 230°C/450°F/Gas Mark 8. Line a baking sheet with non-stick baking parchment.

- Separate the eggs and put the whites into a large clean bowl. Add a pinch of salt. Whisk until the eggs become foamy and thick. Stop when the mixture doesn't move around in the bowl any more and the mixture stands in soft peaks. Scatter over half the chives.

- Spoon half of the beaten whites onto one half of the parchment and spread out so it measures roughly 12cm round. Push the back of the spoon into the middle to create a hollow for the yolk once the whites have baked. Do the same with the other half so you have two mounds of beaten whites.

- Bake in the oven for around 5 minutes. Spoon the egg yolks into the hollows and bake for 3 more minutes until just set. The yolk will still be runny.

- Meanwhile, spread the cream cheese thinly over the rye bread slices. Arrange the smoked salmon on top and scatter over the remaining chives. Season with black pepper and cut each slice in half. Divide between two plates, add the eggs and serve.

Wholesome green smoothie

This low GI smoothie is very green but the sweetness of the apple or pear, the avocado, the honey and coconut water give it a lift which works wonders combined with the kale (which is great for magnesium). Seeds always boost magnesium too, while the good fats in avocado help give skin a genuine glow.

(V) GF **SERVES 1**   273 calories

50g kale or broccoli florets, chopped
½ apple or pear, roughly chopped
¼ avocado, chopped
Good pinch cayenne pepper
50g plain live yoghurt (or a dairy-free alternative
    such as coconut milk yoghurt)

1 tbsp toasted pumpkin or sunflower seeds
100–150ml coconut water or water
1 tsp honey, to sweeten (optional)

- Put the kale or broccoli into a bowl and pour over enough boiling water to cover. Leave for 1–2 minutes, then drain well.

- Put into the bowl of a mini blender or food processor and add the apple or pear, avocado, cayenne, yoghurt and seeds. Blend until smooth. Add the coconut water or water and blend again to combine everything. If you're using the honey, add it now and quickly whizz again.

- Pour into a glass and serve.

LIZ'S TIP

You can also make this the night before you want to enjoy it. Pour into a sealable container and chill.

Nutty granola

This granola can be stored for two weeks but in my house never lasts that long. There are only natural sugars in this rich, nutty recipe, which uses spelt and oat flakes to enhance fibre intake and help reduce cholesterol. Three varieties of nuts will boost vitamin D, protein and calcium – plus provide good fats which will keep you feeling fuller for longer. Tempting as it may be to go back for more, aim for one tea cup-sized portion of this granola to keep the healthy benefits.

(V) MAKES AROUND 400g   228 calories per 40g serving

25g coconut oil	50g oats
50g brazil nuts, chopped	1 egg white
100g whole almonds, chopped	40g date syrup
100g cashew nuts, chopped	1 tsp ground cinnamon
50g spelt flakes	25g coconut flakes

- Preheat the oven to 200°C/400°F/Gas Mark 6. Line a large roasting tin with non-stick baking parchment.

- Spoon the oil onto the parchment then add the nuts, spelt flakes and oats and put the tin in the oven for a minute or two until the coconut oil melts. Give the mixture a good stir so the oil coats the nuts then bake for around 10 minutes. Toss the mixture halfway through and turn the tray round if the nuts are toasting more on one side.

- Whisk the egg white, date syrup and cinnamon together in a bowl until the mixture is slightly paler in colour and looks frothy.

- Add the coconut flakes to the roasting tin, then stir in the egg white mix, too. Continue to bake for 8–12 minutes until the mixture looks slightly crispy and the mixture has started to clump together.

- Cool in the tin then break up and store in a jar for up to 2 weeks.

Three-seed porridge

To pack a protein punch at breakfast there's nothing easier than eating porridge – and nothing simpler than making it yourself. Rich in manganese and a good source of calcium and fibre, oats are low GI so help to keep blood sugar levels steady. Flax seeds (linseeds) are a good source of phytoestrogens, so may help with hormonal hot flushes.

The following ingredients make enough for 10 single portions or five double portions.

Keep the oats and seeds in separate containers, then scoop out and weigh the mix as you need it.

For the porridge mix:
400g oats
40g sunflower seeds

30g flax seeds
30g chia seeds

- Weigh the oats into one jar and seal. Then mix together the seeds and put in a separate jar.

ⓥ SERVES 2   271 calories

80g oats
20g seed mix
¼ tsp ground cinnamon, plus extra to sprinkle

1 greenish banana, chopped
2 tbsp plain live Greek yoghurt

- Put the oats in a pan and add the seed mix, cinnamon and banana. Pour in 450ml water and, stirring constantly, bring to a gentle simmer. Cook for 3–5 minutes, stirring all the time, until the mixture is more or less smooth.

- Spoon between two bowls, top with the Greek yoghurt and sprinkle over a little extra cinnamon.

LIZ'S TIP

If you like, you can soak the oats and seeds the night before. Put into a bowl and pour over 150ml water, cover and set aside. The next day, spoon into a pan and add the remaining 300ml of water and cook as above. Depending on how you like the texture of your porridge, you may need to add more water at this stage.

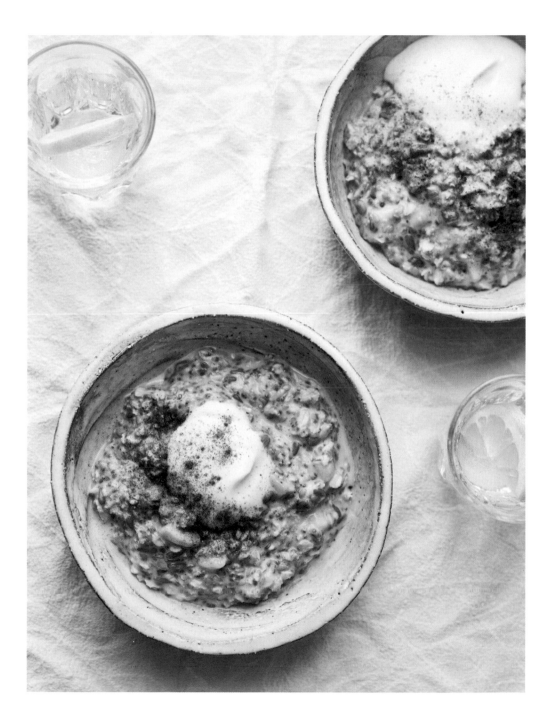

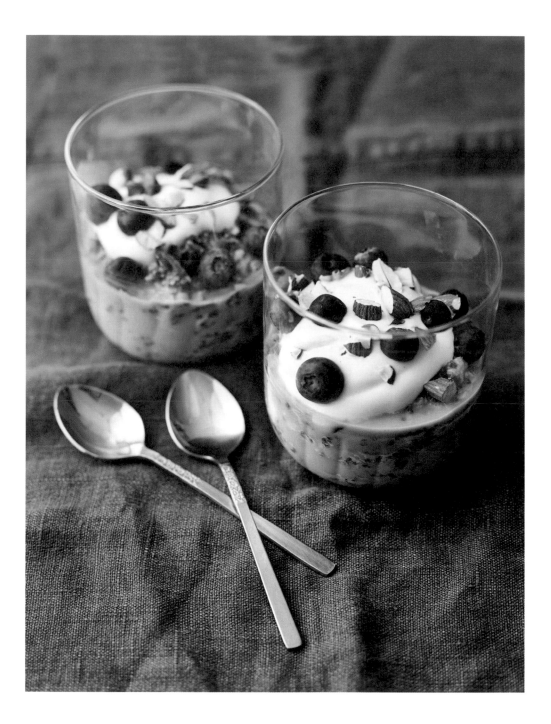

Apple and cinnamon chia pots

I'm always on the lookout for delicious breakfast ideas which double up as late afternoon snacks and this fits the bill. These little pots will keep you feeling full and satisfy any sweet cravings thanks to the cinnamon. There's plenty of fibre in the apples and oats, while the almonds, milk and yoghurt give a good portion of calcium. Chia seeds are full of magnesium, which boosts energy and helps with anxiety and digestion, so do sprinkle liberally!

Ⓥ SERVES 2   227 calories

2 medium apples, grated   ½ tsp ground cinnamon
2 tbsp chia seeds   2 tbsp plain live yoghurt or coconut milk yoghurt
2 tbsp oats   100g blueberries
200ml milk (dairy, oat or nut)   10g whole almonds, chopped

- Put the grated apples in a bowl and add the chia seeds, oats, milk and cinnamon. Stir everything together.

- Divide between two glasses and chill overnight.

- The next day, take the pots out of the fridge, top with the yoghurt and blueberries, then sprinkle over the almonds.

SNACKS

Pistachio, fig, coconut and cacao nib balls

My friends all adore these indulgent treats – as do my family – and we always manage to have more than just one even though they are incredibly rich. Almonds are a good source of protein and calcium, and flax seeds (linseeds) are a vegetarian source of Omega-3 as well as containing phytoestrogens.

V DF GF MAKES 18   64 calories

2–3 dried figs, chopped
100g pistachios
25g whole almonds
1 tbsp flax seeds

2 tsp cacao nibs
1 tbsp soya flour, toasted
2 tbsp unsweetened desiccated coconut

- Put the figs in a bowl and pour over 50ml boiling water. Scatter the pistachios, almonds and flax seeds on top and set aside to soak for 30 minutes.

- Spoon the mixture into a food processor and add the cacao nibs and soya flour. Blitz until the nuts are chopped up and the mixture looks like a pulp. Press a little bit between your fingers to check it will stick together.

- Scoop up heaped teaspoonfuls of the mixture and roll into balls to make around 18 bite-size rounds.

- Put the coconut on a plate and roll the balls in it until coated. Place on a clean plate and chill for 1 hour until firm. Store in an airtight container for up to 5 days or freeze for up to a month.

LIZ'S TIP

Rolling the balls is a bit of a sticky affair so, if you like, you can chill them once made and before rolling in the coconut so that they firm up a little. If you find the desiccated coconut doesn't stick to them as well, roll them in a little cold water first.

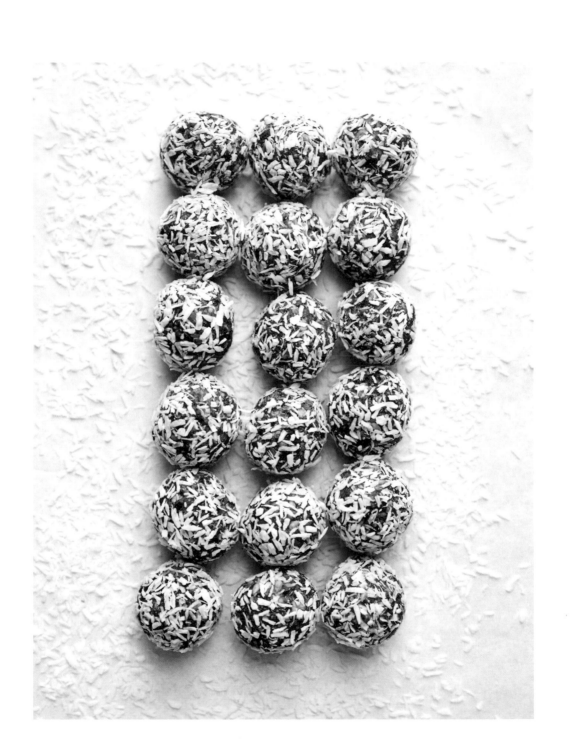

Seeded oatcakes

I keep a tin of these delicious oatcakes in the kitchen at all times – everyone in my family seeks them out as a snack and they are so much better than most shop-bought versions. High in fibre and protein thanks to the seeds and soya flour, these oatcakes are low GI so will not interfere with blood sugar levels.

(V) (DF) MAKES 20   39 calories

50g oats
20g soya flour
1 tbsp flax seeds
1 tbsp sunflower seeds
25g spelt flour

25g wheatgerm
¼ tsp sea salt
2 tbsp olive oil
1 tsp raw organic honey

- Preheat the oven to 200°C/400°F/Gas Mark 6.

- Put the oats, soya flour, flax seeds, sunflower seeds, spelt flour, wheat germ and salt into the bowl of a food processor and whizz briefly to chop up the oats and nuts.

- Add the oil, honey and 4 tablespoons water and whizz again until the mixture just comes together – it should look like a rough dough.

- Tip out onto a piece of baking parchment and press down. Cover with a separate piece of parchment and roll until the mixture is about 3mm thick. Take off the top piece of parchment and use this to line a baking sheet.

- Stamp out rounds with a 5cm cutter. Reroll the end bits of dough and stamp out the remaining rounds until you have 20 biscuits. Spread the biscuits out on the baking sheet and cook for 12–15 minutes until golden.

- Cool on a wire rack and store in an airtight container for up to 5 days.

LIZ'S TIP

These oatcakes freeze well. Wrap tightly in cling film and freeze for up to 1 month. Take one or two out as you fancy.

Liz's snack pots

Goat's cheese and herb pot

Goat's cheese provides plenty of bone-boosting calcium and good fats.

(V) (DF)   150 calories

75g soft goat's cheese
2 tbsp freshly chopped herbs, such as chives and
    parsley
¼ tsp cayenne pepper
Freshly ground black pepper

To serve:
Crudités – 1 small chopped carrot, 1 chopped
    celery stalk, 3–4 each radishes and cherry
    tomatoes, quartered

- Spoon the goat's cheese into a bowl and beat in the herbs, cayenne and black pepper. If the mixture is very thick and you prefer the dip to be softer, stir in 1–2 teaspoons water.

- Divide between two plates and serve with the crudités to dip into.

Strawberry yoghurt pot

Packed with vitamin C and calcium, my children love the bright red of this yoghurt which lets the natural sweetness of the strawberries and syrup or honey shine through.

(V) (DF)   102 calories

150g ripe strawberries, chopped
1 tsp balsamic vinegar

1 tsp date syrup or honey
6 tbsp plain live Greek yoghurt

- Put the strawberries, vinegar and syrup or honey into a bowl and mash with a fork until half the strawberries have broken down and are like a pulp. Spoon the yoghurt into the bowl and fold together – the strawberry mixture should be marbled through the yoghurt.

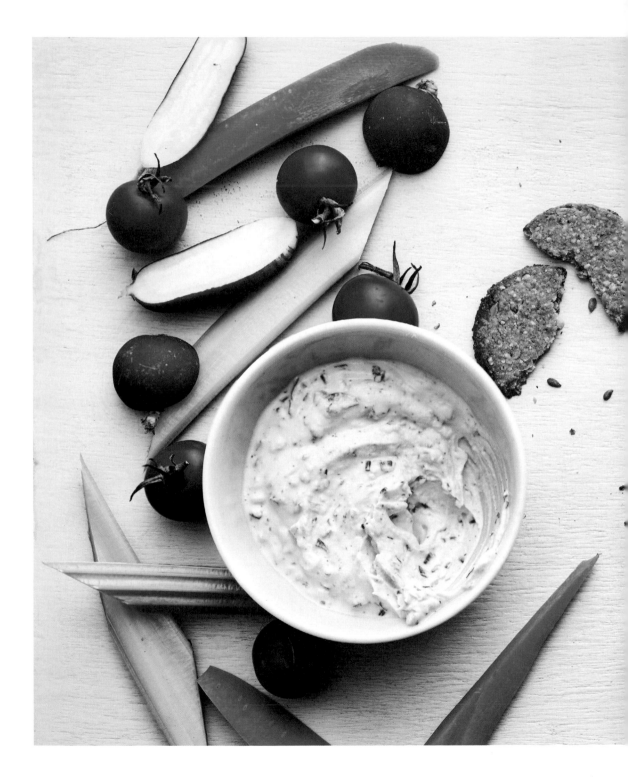

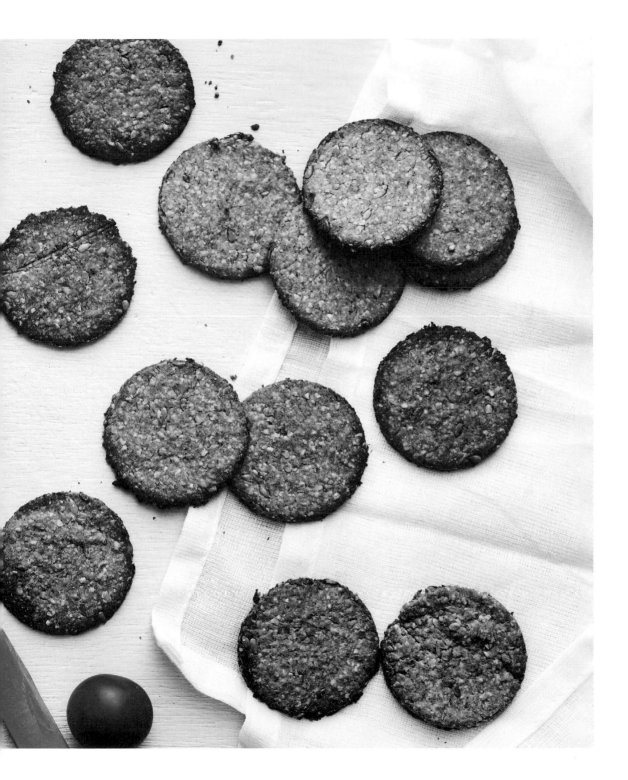

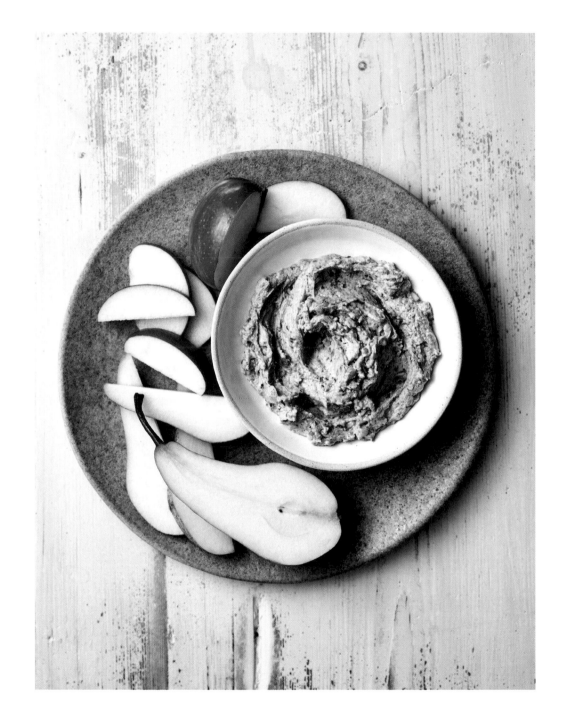

Nut butter pot

I love this light and delicious spread packed with protein from the nuts, which will keep you full until supper. Cinnamon helps to curb cravings for a biscuit, while live yoghurt boasts calcium and gut-friendly probiotics.

(V) (DF)   193 calories

2 tbsp nut butter, such as peanut or almond
½ tsp ground cinnamon
3 tbsp plain live yoghurt

To serve:
1 each pear and apple, sliced, including pips and
    core

- Put the butter, cinnamon and yoghurt into a bowl and mix all the ingredients together. You may want to add a teaspoon of water to loosen it if needed.

- Divide between two plates. Arrange half the apple and pear slices on each.

Fresh figs and cottage cheese

Fresh figs may be an aphrodisiac but they're also packed with much-needed calcium, magnesium and fibre. Offset the natural sweetness with plain organic cottage cheese (a good source of protein), while brazil nuts will add to your selenium intake for the day.

V GF **SERVES 2**   129 calories

4 fresh figs
4 tbsp cottage cheese or ricotta

4 brazil nuts, chopped
½ tsp honey or date syrup (optional)

- Split the figs through the middle, then arrange on two plates.

- Put the cottage cheese or ricotta in a bowl and fold in half the brazil nuts.

- Spoon among the figs, scatter over the remaining nuts and drizzle with honey or date syrup, if using.

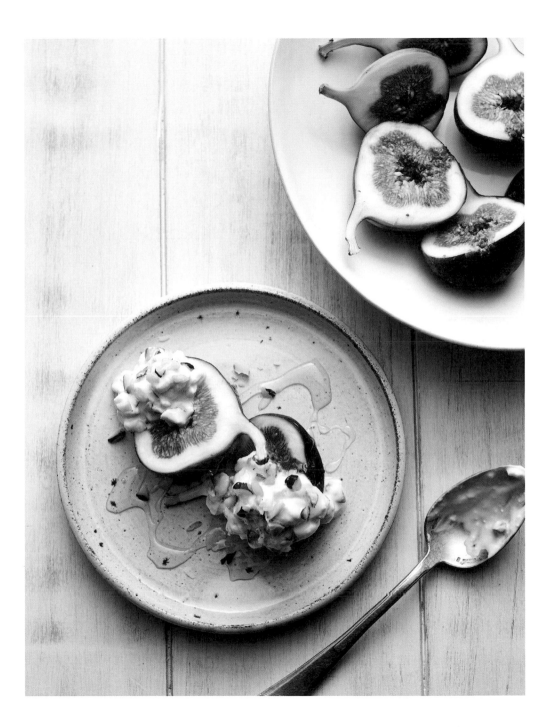

LIGHT MEALS

Cauliflower Steaks with hummus and feta

As long as you don't overcook the cauli it is a great source of vitamin C and is delicious topped with creamy hummus made from chickpeas, which are packed with fibre, protein and phytoestrogens. Feta is made from goat's or sheep's milk and is an ideal non-dairy source of protein.

V GF SERVES 2   387 calories

½ x 400g can chickpeas, drained
1 tbsp tahini
Juice of ½ lemon
Sea salt and freshly ground black pepper
1 medium cauliflower
1 tsp olive oil
Pinch cayenne pepper
50g feta cheese, crumbled
1 tbsp mixed toasted seeds

For the tomato salad:
150g mixed tomatoes (red, yellow and heritage), quartered
1 tsp cider vinegar
Sprig of basil, roughly chopped
sea salt and freshly ground black pepper

- Preheat the grill.

- First make the salad. Put the tomatoes, vinegar and basil in a bowl and season. Mix together. The juices from the tomatoes will make a natural dressing.

- Put the chickpeas, tahini and lemon juice into a small blender or food processor and season. Whizz until the chickpeas have broken down but the mixture is still quite chunky. Season well and whizz again.

- Use a sharp knife to slice the cauliflower into 4 thick 'steaks' from the middle (use the leftover pieces for cauliflower rice – see page 176). Mix the oil and cayenne together, brush the steaks with the dressing and season well. Place the steaks on a baking sheet and grill for 2–3 minutes until golden. Turn over and grill on the other side.

- Arrange 2 steaks on each plate. Spoon the hummus on top, scatter over the feta and seeds and serve with the tomato salad.

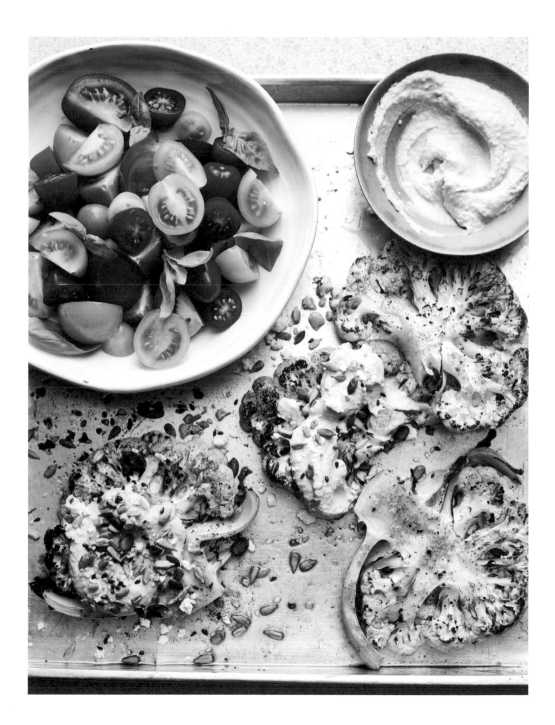

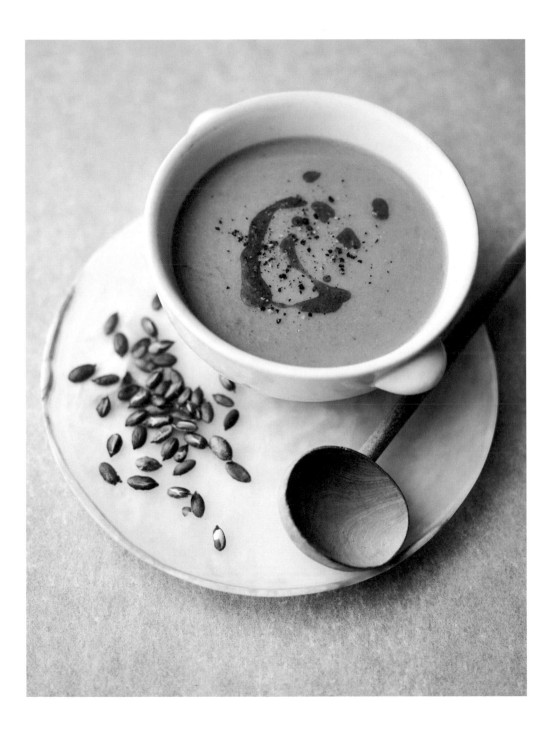

Carrot and squash soup with rocket drizzle

My warming winter soup gives a gorgeous orange glow from the carrots which are packed with antioxidants and vitamin B, and garlic boosts the immune system. I like to include squash as, besides adding vitamin C and magnesium, it imparts a subtle sweet flavour. I sprinkle toasted pumpkin seeds on soups as they're rich in monounsaturated fatty acids which can help to lower bad cholesterol and increase good cholesterol.

(V) (DF) MAKES 4 PORTIONS   232 calories

1 tbsp olive oil

1 red onion, roughly chopped

2 carrots, chopped

250g squash, chopped (no need to peel if
   the skin is soft)

½ red chilli, deseeded and chopped

1 clove garlic, sliced

Sea salt and freshly ground black pepper

600ml hot vegetable stock

1 tbsp toasted pumpkin seeds, to serve

For the drizzle:

40g rocket

75ml olive oil

- Heat the oil in a medium pan and add the onion, carrots and squash and a tablespoon of water. Sauté over a low to medium heat for 10 minutes until the vegetables start to soften.

- Stir in the chilli and garlic and cook for 2–3 minutes more. Season. Pour in the hot stock, cover the pan with a lid and bring to a simmer. Cook for 12–15 minutes or until tender.

- Meanwhile, whizz the rocket and oil together in a mini blender.

- Allow the soup to cool a little, then purée with a stick blender. Spoon half the soup into a sealable container and set aside to cool completely before freezing (see tip).

- Divide the remaining soup between two bowls, top with the rocket drizzle and serve scattered with the pumpkin seeds.

LIZ'S TIP

This soup freezes well. Freeze for up to 3 months, then thaw overnight at a cool room temperature. Reheat and finish the soup as above.

Warm beetroot rice and lentil salad with mackerel

Strong but subtle flavours make this low GI lunch packed with Omega-3s from the mackerel a filling dish. Beetroot offers liver support and is a potent blood booster too, while walnuts provide a dose of calcium and healthy fats.

DF **GF** **SERVES 2** 617 calories

2–4 mackerel fillets (around 300g), depending on how large they are

Oil, for brushing

For the beetroot and lentil salad:
125g beetroot, peeled and roughly chopped
1 tbsp red wine vinegar
1 tbsp olive oil

Sea salt and freshly ground black pepper
75g dried puy lentils
1 tbsp finely chopped chives
½ tsp Dijon mustard, plus extra to serve
20g toasted walnuts, chopped
Juice of ½ lemon
Small handful of watercress, to serve

- Tip the beetroot into a food processor and blitz until the pieces resemble rice. Spoon into a bowl and stir in the vinegar and oil. Season well, stir again and set aside.

- Put the lentils into a pan and cover with plenty of cold water. Cover with a lid and bring to the boil. Turn the heat down low and simmer for 20–25 minutes until tender. Drain well.

- Spoon the beetroot mixture, along with any marinade, into the lentils and keep warm.

- Preheat the grill. Brush the mackerel with oil and lay flat, skin side down, on a baking sheet. Grill for 5–6 minutes until the fish is cooked through.

- Stir the chives, mustard, walnuts and lemon juice into the lentil mixture and divide between two plates. Top with the mackerel and serve with the watercress and some mustard on the side.

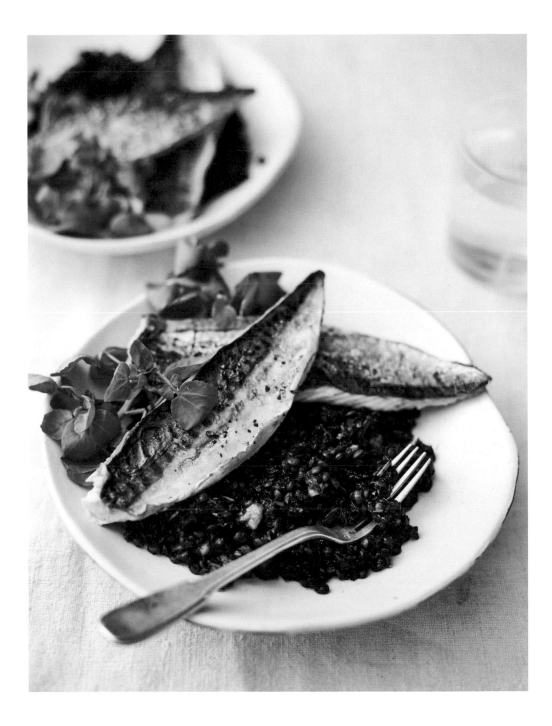

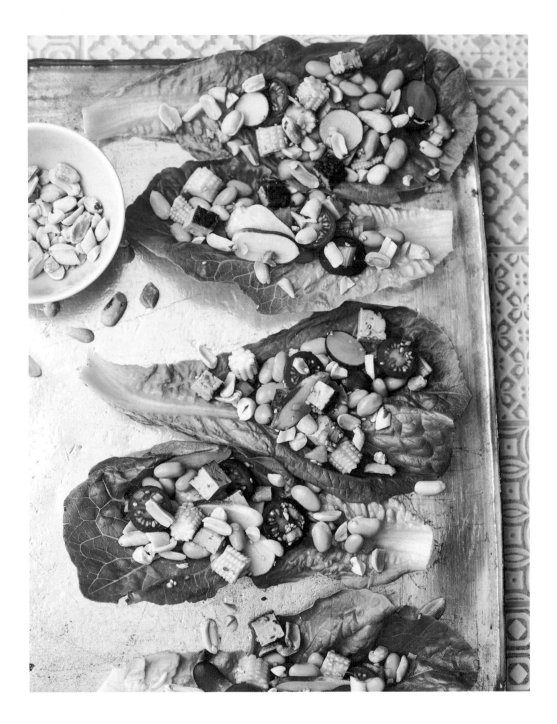

Tempeh wraps

These wraps look so inviting and make for a nutritious alternative to a lunch sandwich, using proteins other than meat, fish or dairy. I love soya beans for their iron content, protein and phytoestrogens, while tempeh, sweetcorn and peanuts offer plenty of protein.

V DF SERVES 2   319 calories

1 tbsp cider vinegar
1 shallot, finely chopped
100g frozen soya beans, thawed
2 stalks celery, finely chopped
50g baby sweetcorn, chopped
75g radishes, chopped
75g cherry tomatoes, chopped
75g tempeh or smoked tofu, chopped
8 large cos lettuce leaves
20g toasted peanuts, chopped

For the dressing:
1 tbsp sesame oil
1 tbsp soy sauce
Juice of 1 lime
½ tbsp toasted sesame seeds
¼ tsp ground white pepper

- Whisk all the ingredients for the dressing in a bowl then set aside.

- Put the vinegar and shallot in a large bowl and set aside for 10 minutes – this softens the sharpness of the shallot. Strain, leaving the marinated shallots in the bowl. Add the soya beans, celery, sweetcorn, radishes, tomatoes, tempeh or smoked tofu and stir to mix.

- Arrange the lettuce leaves on a large platter. Pour the dressing over the vegetable salad and mix everything together. Spoon the salad into the lettuce wraps, sprinkle over the peanuts and enjoy.

Summer minestrone

I love this light summer soup which retains the freshness of all the veggie ingredients. Fennel aids digestion, peas are an unlikely source of protein and asparagus is a very gut-healthy prebiotic as well as containing chromium, a mineral which helps insulin carry glucose from the bloodstream into the cells.

Ⓥ MAKES 4 PORTIONS   176 calories

1 tbsp olive oil
2 shallots, chopped
2 stalks celery, diced
1 carrot, diced
Sea salt and freshly ground black pepper
50g farro
800ml hot vegetable or chicken stock

½ fennel bulb, chopped
150g asparagus tips, chopped
100g podded peas
100g thawed soya beans
2 sprigs of basil, roughly chopped
Pecorino cheese, to serve

- Heat the oil in a medium pan and stir in the shallots, celery and carrot. Add a tablespoon of water and season well. Cover the pan with a lid, turn the heat down low and simmer for 10 minutes or until the vegetables start to soften. Make sure they don't colour during this time.

- Add the farro and stock and bring to a simmer. Cook for around 25 minutes or until just tender.

- Stir in the fennel, asparagus, peas and soya beans and cook for a further 3–5 minutes until the vegetables have poached in the stock.

- Pour half into a sealable container to chill (see tip).

- Divide the remaining soup between two bowls, scatter over the basil and serve with pecorino to grate over the top.

LIZ'S TIP

This soup will keep in the fridge for up to 4 days. Cool the soup down in the container, then transfer to the fridge. You can either reheat in a pan until hot or it's very nice served chilled, too, with a spoonful of ricotta and a drizzle of extra virgin olive oil on top.

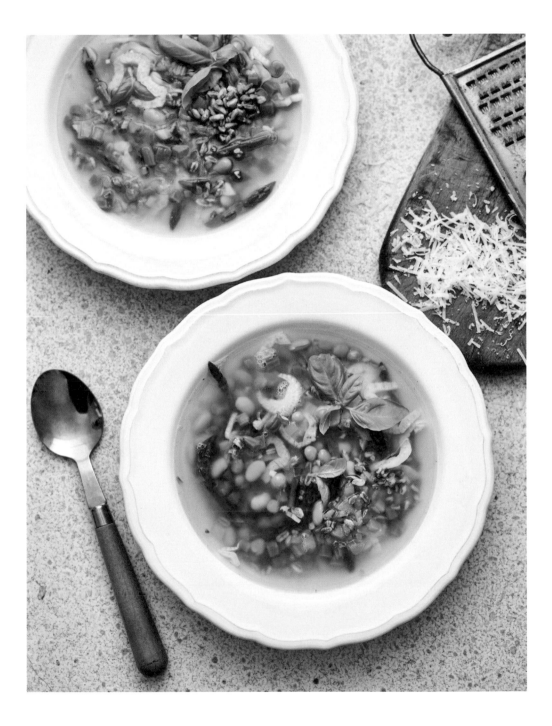

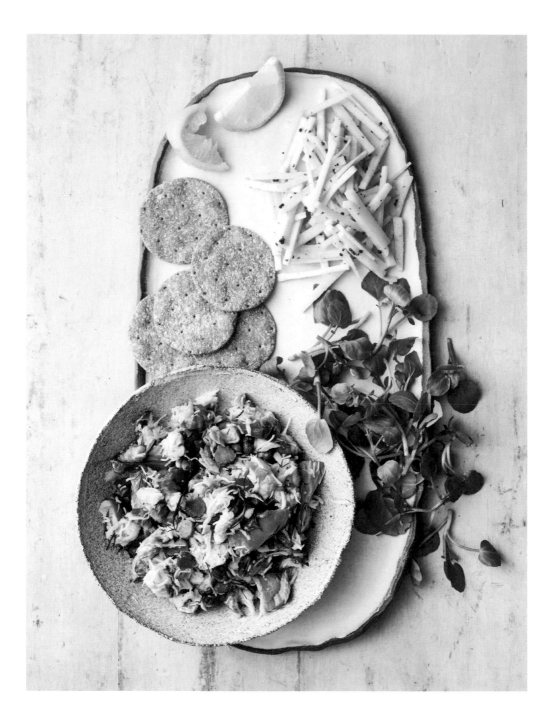

Celeriac and kohlrabi remoulade with seafood

I serve this very pretty-looking starter with crackers as it is quite rich – the wonderful seafood gives all the Omega-3s and protein you will need even before the main course! Mild-flavoured celeriac is full of fibre and offers vitamins B6 and B5, while kohlrabi provides vitamin C.

DF SERVES 2   520 calories

For the remoulade:
1 large egg yolk
1 tbsp boiling water
35ml olive oil
1 tsp wholegrain mustard
1 tsp cider vinegar
Sea salt and freshly ground black pepper
200g celeriac, peeled and cut into matchsticks
160g kohlrabi, peeled and cut into matchsticks

For the seafood:
250g mixed cured fish, such as crayfish, crab, hot
    smoked trout or salmon
3 cornichon gherkins, chopped
2 tbsp freshly chopped dill
1 tbsp non-pareil capers

To serve:
Small handful of watercress or rocket
4 wholewheat crackers
½ lemon, halved

- Whisk the egg yolk, boiling water, olive oil, mustard and vinegar together in a large bowl and season well. Add the celeriac and kohlrabi and toss to mix.

- Put the cured fish in a separate bowl – flake the fish if you're using smoked trout or salmon as it needs to be broken up. Add the gherkins, dill, capers and 1–2 teaspoons of the juice from the jar of capers and toss together to mix everything evenly.

- Divide the remoulade and seafood between two plates, dress with the watercress or rocket and serve with the crackers and a lemon wedge to squeeze over.

Saucy butter beans with dill

This is my grown-up, healthy version of egg and baked beans. It has plenty of intense colour from the cooked tomatoes, which contain lycopene, and provides protein and, of course, fibre which, if eaten for a light lunch, will keep you full until dinner.

Ⓥ ⒹⒻ SERVES 2   237 calories

1 tbsp olive oil

½ small onion, finely chopped

1 stalk celery, finely chopped

2 cloves garlic, sliced

½ x 400g can chopped tomatoes

1 tsp tomato purée

100ml hot vegetable stock

Sea salt and freshly ground black pepper

2 tbsp freshly chopped dill, plus a few sprigs to garnish

400g can butter beans, drained well

2 medium eggs

- Heat the oil in a pan and cook the onion, celery and garlic over a low heat for 10–15 minutes.

- Meanwhile, bring a medium pan of water to a simmer.

- Stir the chopped tomatoes, tomato purée and stock into the pan with the vegetables, then season well and bring to a simmer. Cook for 10 minutes, uncovered, to thicken slightly. Whizz with a stick blender until smooth, then stir in the dill and drained beans. Add 2–3 tablespoons water if the mixture is very thick and cook for 2–3 minutes more to heat through.

- Poach the eggs. Turn the heat in the pan of water down to low, so the water is just simmering. Carefully drop each egg into it, spaced apart. Cook for around 3 minutes. Lift both eggs out with a slotted spoon and drain on kitchen paper.

- Divide the beans between two plates, top with an egg and serve garnished with a few sprigs of dill.

LIZ'S TIP

Great on a slice of lightly buttered sourdough. Alternatively, serve with a handful of steamed green beans or a green salad on the side.

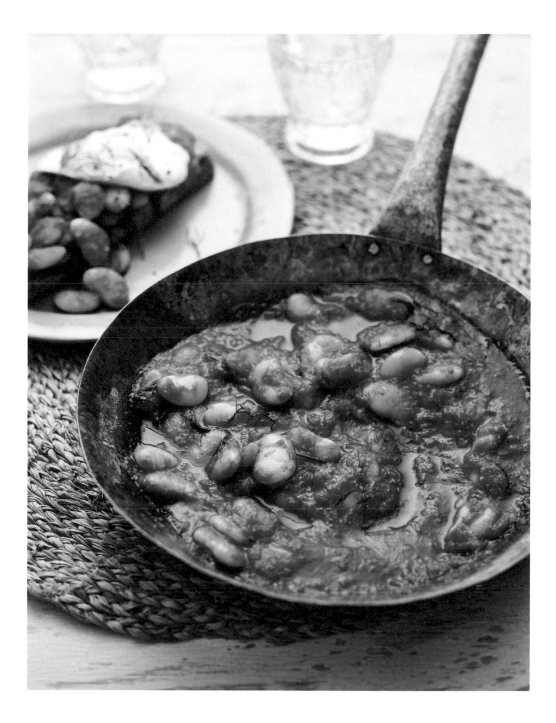

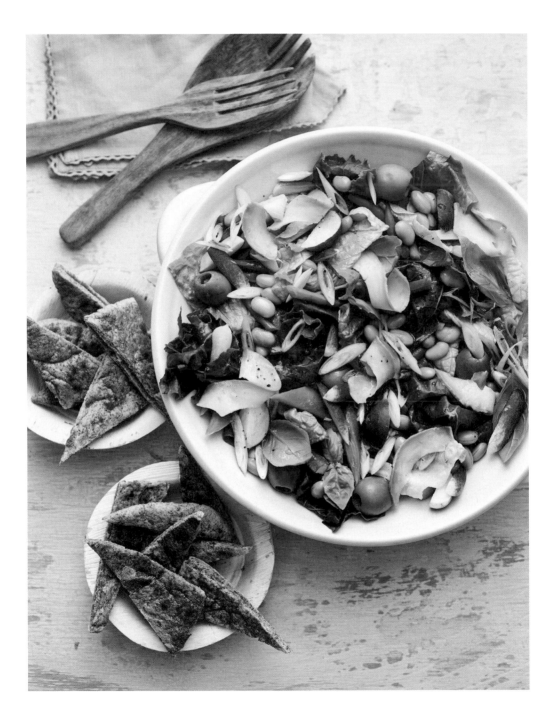

Warm green bean salad

This luscious-looking green salad packs a powerful punch when it comes to meno-healthy nutrients. Combining the crunch of the beans and spring onions with the smoothness of the avocado (Omega-3s and prebiotics), plus protein from the soya beans, olives and olive oil, the dish is then topped off with basil and its excellent anti-inflammatory properties.

Ⓥ ⒹⒻ SERVES 2   331 calories

100g green beans, chopped into 3cm chunks

100g runner beans, chopped into 2–3cm chunks

70g frozen soya beans

50g kale, roughly torn

2 spring onions, roughly chopped

½ romaine lettuce, roughly chopped

4–6 radishes, quartered lengthways

½ avocado, sliced

6 large green olives

2 sprigs of basil, finely chopped

1 tbsp extra virgin olive oil

1 tbsp red, white or cider vinegar

Sea salt and freshly ground black pepper

For the pitta crisps:

1 wholemeal pitta

A little oil, for brushing

Cayenne pepper, to sprinkle

- Bring a large pan of water to the boil and cook the green beans, runner beans and soya beans for 4–5 minutes or until tender. Add the kale and spring onions, then drain well in a sieve.

- Put the lettuce into a large salad bowl. Add the radishes, avocado, olives and basil. Whisk together the oil and vinegar in a separate bowl and season well. Pour over the lettuce mix then add the cooked greens and toss everything together.

- Toast the pitta, then cut into triangles. Brush each triangle with a little oil and season, then sprinkle lightly with cayenne. Serve with the salad.

LIZ'S TIP

This is a wholesome dish as it stands, but if you have any tofu, it works brilliantly in this salad, too. I like the flavoured tofus, such as olive, which goes perfectly with the other ingredients in here. Just finely chop 75–100g tofu and scatter over the top of the salad before serving.

Five-veg fritters

Eating vegetables needn't be dull! The vibrant colours of these fritters make for a wonderfully bright plate and, of course, colours equal antioxidants, so they're great for overall health too. The eggs make sure this meal supplies enough protein, while soya flour boosts the phytoestrogen, iron and magnesium content.

V DF GF **SERVES 2**   332 calories

½ courgette, roughly chopped

½ medium carrot, roughly chopped

1 spring onion, roughly chopped

½ red pepper, deseeded and roughly chopped

2 medium eggs

4 tbsp soya flour

Good pinch cayenne pepper

4 tbsp sweetcorn (fresh from a cob or canned)

2 tbsp freshly chopped herbs, such as parsley, chives and basil

Sea salt and freshly ground black pepper

1–2 tbsp olive oil

- Put the courgette, carrot, spring onion and red pepper into the bowl of a food processor and blitz until the vegetables are finely chopped and look a little like rice.

- Beat the eggs, soya flour and cayenne together in a bowl. Add the chopped vegetables, sweetcorn and herbs and season well. Fold everything together until the mixture is combined.

- Heat the oil in a large frying pan until just hot. Use a tablespoon to scoop up the mixture and place 4–5 dollops in the pan, spacing them well apart.

- Cook until the mixture looks as though it is just starting to set, and the fritters are golden underneath, then flip over and cook the other side until set. Lift out and put on a plate and continue to cook the mixture until it's all used up.

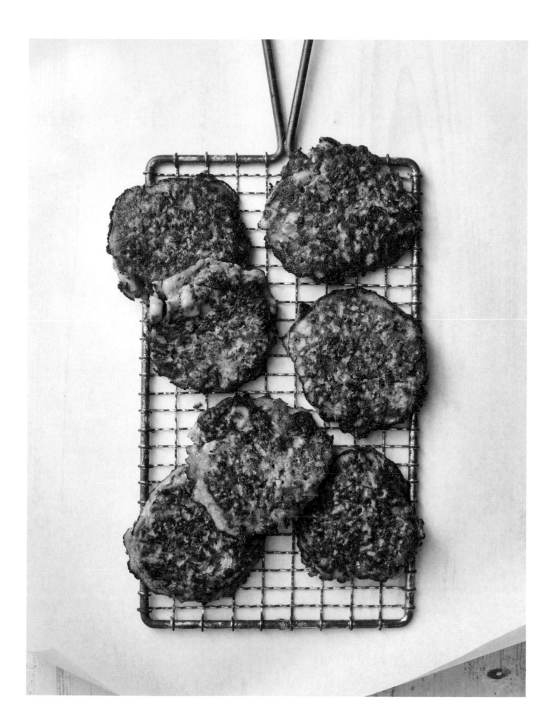

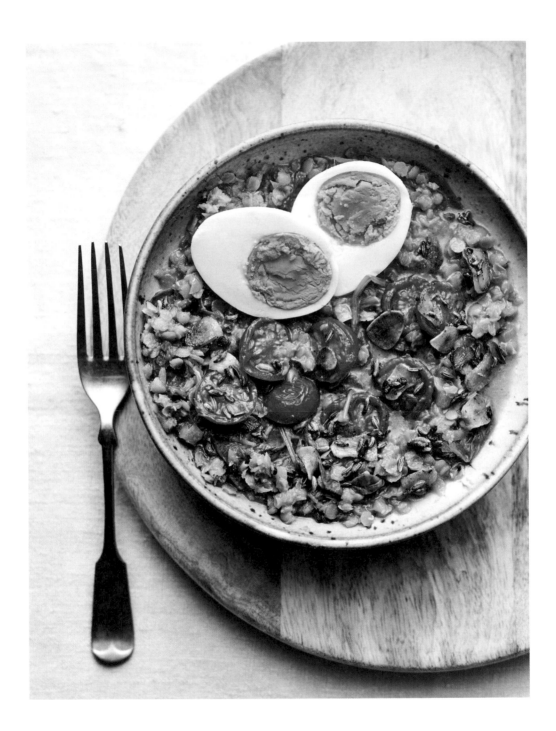

Red lentil, spinach, tomato and egg curry with ghee

This bright, robust curry is a real treat of taste and colour. There's nothing like lentils for an excellent source of protein (that goes for the eggs too), B vitamins and fibre. Tomatoes give a boost of lycopene, turmeric and cumin have anti-inflammatory properties, while garlic supports the immune system.

(V) (DF) SERVES 2   432 calories

2 large eggs	Sea salt and freshly ground black pepper
30g ghee	100g dried red lentils
½ small onion, finely chopped	600ml hot vegetable stock
1 tsp turmeric	2 cloves garlic, sliced
1 tsp ground coriander	8 cherry tomatoes, halved
1 tsp ground cumin	1 tsp cumin seeds
Good pinch chilli powder (omit if you find this causes hot flushes)	100g baby spinach leaves

- Put the eggs in a small pan and cover with cold water. Bring to the boil and simmer for 8 minutes. Lift the eggs out and transfer to a bowl of cold water to cool.

- Heat half the ghee in a saucepan and stir-fry the onion over a medium heat for 8–10 minutes until starting to turn golden. Stir in the spices, along with 2 tablespoons water, and cook, stirring the ingredients, until the water has evaporated. Season well.

- Stir in the lentils and stock, cover the pan with a lid and turn the heat down low. Cook for 15–20 minutes, stirring every now and then, until the lentils have softened.

- Meanwhile, peel and halve the eggs.

- About 5 minutes before the end of cooking, heat the remaining ghee in a frying pan and stir in the garlic, tomatoes and cumin seeds. Cook until the garlic turns golden and the tomatoes have softened.

- Stir the spinach into the lentils then divide between two bowls. Spoon over the garlic, cherry tomato and cumin mix then arrange the eggs on top.

Nori wrap bites

Like many delicious vegetarian dishes there's a lot of chopping involved – but it's always worth it for the taste! Nori seaweed is a great bone booster as it's high in vitamin C, calcium and magnesium, while carrots add silica. Besides the abundant protein in chickpeas, these wraps are packed with phytoestrogens thanks to the sesame seeds.

(V) (DF) GF SERVES 2   152 calories

For the chickpea and pepper spread:
½ x 400g can chickpeas, drained
1 marinated red pepper, drained well
½ lemon, halved
Sea salt and freshly ground black pepper

For the bites:
2 square sheets nori seaweed
6–8 cos lettuce leaves, each cut into thirds along
    the length
1 small carrot, cut into long matchsticks
¼ cucumber, deseeded and cut into long
    matchsticks
2 spring onions, halved and cut into long
    matchsticks
1 tbsp toasted seeds, such as sesame and pumpkin
    (optional)

- Put the chickpeas into the bowl of a mini food processor or blender. Add the pepper and squeeze over the juice from one of the lemon quarters. Season well. Whizz to make a purée – it can be as chunky or as smooth as you fancy.

- Lay the nori seaweed squares flat on a board and press half the lettuce leaves down on top of each to cover about four-fifths of each square. Top each with half the carrot, cucumber and spring onions and squeeze over the remaining lemon quarter. Season well.

- Roughly spread half the chickpea and pepper purée over the vegetables on each nori square. Sprinkle the seeds on top if you're using them.

- Take the nearest edge of one of the pieces of seaweed and roll up. When you get to the end bit of nori, wet it, then fold it onto the wrap to secure.

- Do the same with the other square of nori so you have two wraps. Slice each in half and serve.

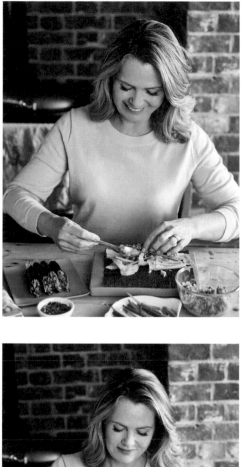

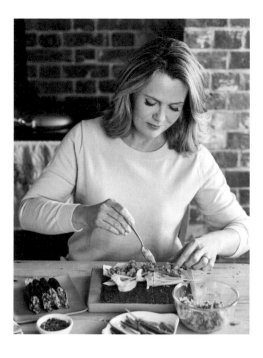

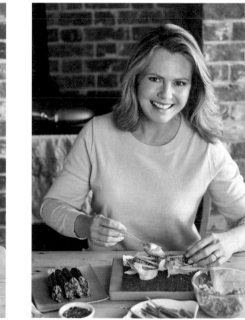

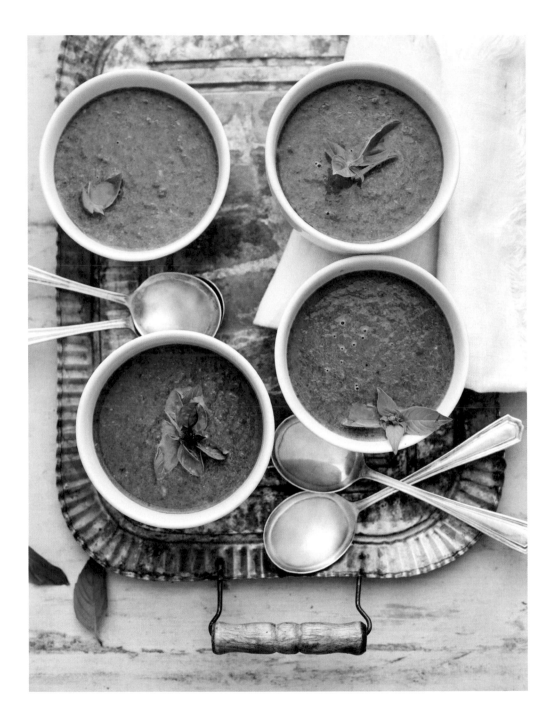

Thai-spiced spinach and watercress soup

Don't worry that this soup will bring you out in a hot flush! My version of watercress soup gives it a spicy twist but the chilli is optional. Spicy watercress is brimming with iron, while spinach offers vitamin C, and the basil, ginger and turmeric are all anti-inflammatory ingredients.

(V) (DF) **MAKES 4 PORTIONS**   62 calories

1 tbsp coconut oil

3 shallots, chopped

5cm fresh ginger (around 30g), peeled and
    chopped

½ tsp turmeric

2 cloves garlic, sliced

1 stalk lemongrass, chopped

½ red or green chilli, chopped (optional)

Sea salt and freshly ground black pepper

260g spinach

80g watercress

600ml hot vegetable stock

Small handful of basil leaves (preferably Thai basil
    if you can get it), plus a few extra to serve

½ lime, halved

- Heat the coconut oil in a pan and stir in the shallots, ginger, turmeric, garlic, lemongrass, chilli and a tablespoon of water. Cook over a low to medium heat for 5 minutes until the ingredients are starting to soften and turn golden. Season well.

- Stir in the spinach and watercress then pour in the stock. Cover the pan with a lid and simmer for around 10 minutes. Turn off the heat. Add the basil leaves, then blend the soup with a heatproof stick blender until smooth.

- Pour half into a freezer-proof container and set aside to cool (you can freeze this for up to 3 months). Divide the soup between two bowls, scatter with the extra basil and serve with a wedge of lime to squeeze over.

LIZ'S TIP

For a creamy coconut-rich flavour, stir in 100ml coconut milk after blitzing the soup and heat through. If you have any leftover roast chicken, you can use it to add extra flavour and texture to this soup. Chop around 100g into small pieces and add to the soup before blitzing, then finish the recipe as above.

Socca pancake

Would you guess this is a vegan dish? Such a wonderful array of spice, flavours and bright veggies offering antioxidants and beta carotene fill these light pancakes made from gram flour – which provides both magnesium and protein.

V DF GF **SERVES 2**   405 calories

75g gram flour

¼ tsp turmeric

Sea salt and freshly ground black pepper

2 tbsp olive oil, plus 1 tsp for frying

½ red onion, thickly sliced

1 tsp ground coriander

1 tsp ground cumin

2 cloves garlic, sliced

½ x 400g can chickpeas, drained

100g asparagus tips

100g purple sprouting or tender-stem broccoli

½ red pepper, deseeded and sliced

50g kale, finely chopped

½ lemon, to squeeze over

- Sift the flour and turmeric, along with a good pinch of salt, into a bowl and make a well in the middle. Gradually pour 150ml water into the middle, whisking constantly. Set aside for 15 minutes while you prepare the topping.

- Heat a tablespoon of the oil in a frying pan and stir-fry the onion for 5 minutes over a medium heat until starting to soften. Stir in the spices, garlic and a tablespoon of water and cook for 1–2 minutes. Add the chickpeas, asparagus, broccoli, pepper and kale and continue to stir-fry for 5 minutes until the vegetables are tender. Season well and cover to keep warm.

- Heat a large frying pan (around 25cm base) until hot. Whisk the remaining tablespoon of oil into the pancake mixture. Put the teaspoon of oil into the frying pan and tip the pan around so that the oil covers the base. Pour the pancake mix into the pan, then lower the heat to low to medium and cook for 5 minutes until the pancake is set. There's no need to flip it, and it should cook until golden and slightly crusty on the bottom.

- Squeeze the lemon juice over the vegetables and stir everything together. Spoon on top of the pancake, cut it in half and and serve.

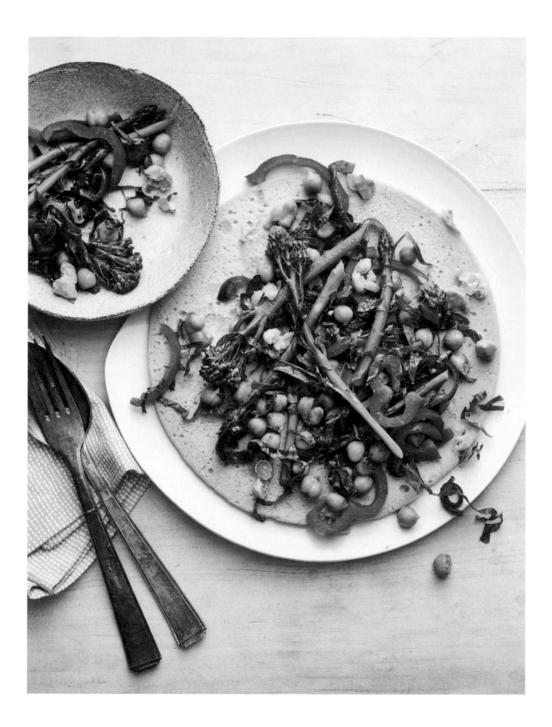

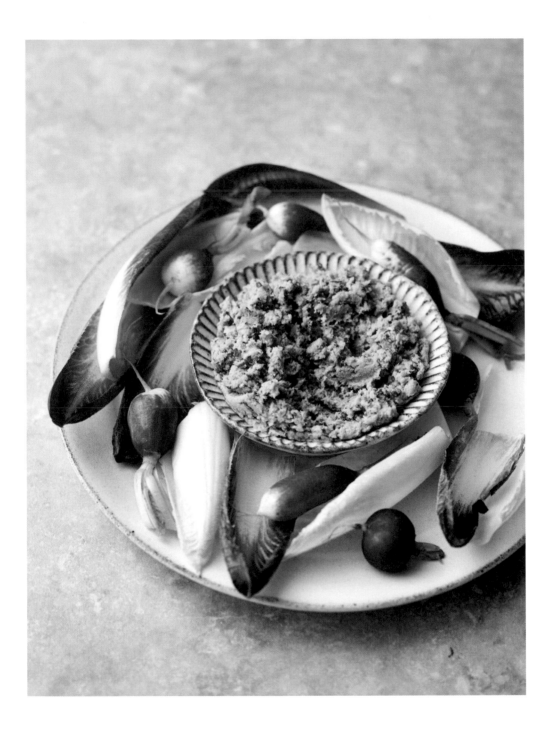

Fresh mackerel pâté

Making your own mackerel pâté really is so simple and the results are far better than anything I have found in a shop. Mackerel is a rich source of Omega-3 fatty acids plus bone-building vitamin D. I like to serve this as a light starter or as a snack – it will keep for 2 days in the fridge.

DF GF SERVES 2, GENEROUSLY   293 calories

2 mackerel fillets (buy them lightly smoked if you can get them)
Sea salt and freshly ground black pepper
1½ tsp wholegrain mustard
1 tbsp olive oil, plus extra for brushing
Juice of ½ lemon

1–2 tbsp freshly chopped Greek basil
1–2 tbsp freshly chopped chives

To serve:
1 chicory bulb
Small handful of radishes

- Brush the mackerel with oil and season well. Grill for 3–4 minutes until the fish has turned opaque and is cooked through. Test with a fork by pushing it into the centre of one of the fillets and pulling a little bit away. If it flakes easily, they're done. Set aside to cool.

- Flake the fish into the bowl of a small food processor, removing the skin and any bones as you do this.

- Add the mustard, olive oil and lemon juice and season well. Pulse the mixture until it comes together into a more or less smooth pâté.

- Pull the chicory leaves away from the bulb and arrange on a plate with the radishes. Spoon the mackerel into two bowls and serve with a sprinkling of herbs.

LIZ'S TIP

You can also pan-fry the mackerel. Brush with oil as above, then cook flesh side down for 3–4 minutes. Turn over and cook on the skin side for 1–2 minutes more or until the fish is cooked through. Complete the recipe as above.

MAIN MEALS

Chicken with lemon and sage

A simple dish that delivers knockout nutrients. Organic chicken breasts provide wonderful lean protein and vitamin B6, which allows the body to use and store energy from protein and carbohydrates. And not only do green beans offer fibre, they're also a source of calcium and iron. Sage is known for helping to calm hot flushes and here adds a delicious fresh flavour.

GF SERVES 2   453 calories

2 skinless organic chicken breasts
1 tbsp olive oil
Juice of ½ lemon
Small sprig of sage, leaves chopped
Sea salt and freshly ground black pepper

2 sweet potatoes (around 350g), unpeeled and
    chopped
15g butter
150g green beans, trimmed

- Lay the chicken breasts on a board and bash with a rolling pin until half the thickness. Transfer to a shallow dish then pour over the oil and lemon juice. Add the chopped sage leaves to the dish and season well. Turn the chicken breasts over so they're completely coated. Set aside.

- Put the sweet potatoes in a pan of water. Cover with a lid and bring to the boil. Once boiling, turn the heat down a little and simmer for 15–20 minutes until soft.

- After the sweet potatoes have been cooking for about 10 minutes, heat a frying pan until hot. Fry the chicken until golden all over and cooked through – it'll take 3–5 minutes on each side. When one side is done, turn over and add the remaining marinade to the pan and continue to cook the other side over a low to medium heat. To check the chicken is cooked through, pierce the middle of one with a sharp knife to make sure there are no pink juices or pink bits left.

- Bring a small pan of water to the boil and simmer the green beans for 3–5 minutes until tender. Drain well, then return to the pan and add half the butter. Set aside for the butter to melt, then season and toss together.

- Drain the sweet potatoes well then return to the pan briefly to steam. Add the remaining butter, season and mash. Spoon onto two plates, followed by the green beans and a chicken breast each. Lastly, drizzle any juices from the pan over the top.

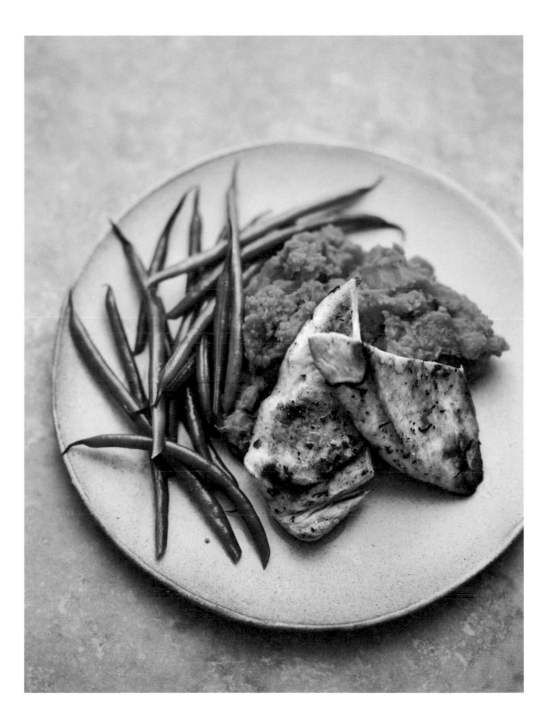

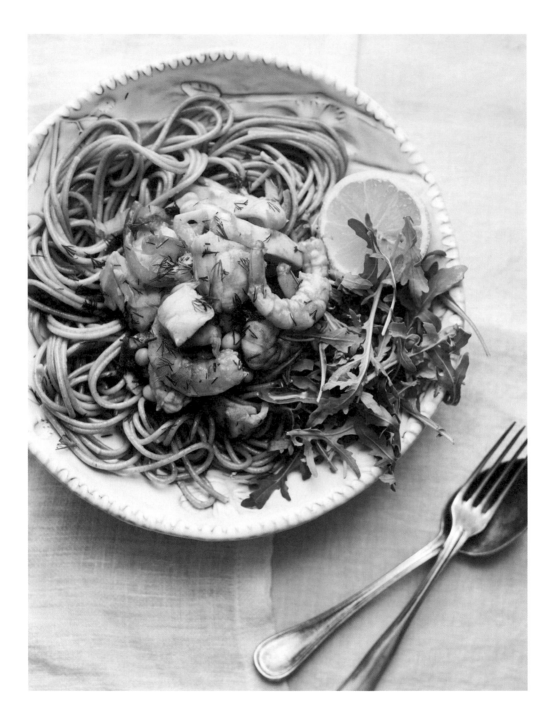

Saturday night seafood feast

Who needs pizza when you can feast on delicious seafood and pasta? The fish provides Omega-3s and plenty of low-fat protein, while cannellini beans add fibre, magnesium and zinc. Should you indulge more than you ought (so easy with this dish!), the fennel aids digestion and gives a hit of vitamin C.

(DF) SERVES 20   592 calories

1 tbsp olive oil, plus extra to drizzle

½ red onion, sliced

2 cloves garlic, sliced

½ fennel bulb, finely chopped

Sea salt and freshly ground black pepper

150g wholewheat spaghetti

½ x 400g can chopped tomatoes

150ml hot light fish or chicken stock

½ x 400g can cannellini beans, drained

250g mixed seafood, such as squid, prawns and cod

1 tbsp freshly chopped dill

Small handful of rocket

½ lemon, halved

- Bring a large pan of water to the boil for the pasta.

- Heat the oil in a medium pan and add a tablespoon of water. Add the onion, garlic and fennel, and season. Cover with a lid and sauté over a low to medium heat for 10–12 minutes, stirring every now and then.

- Cook the pasta according to the packet instructions. Drain well and return to the pan with a drizzle of olive oil.

- Stir the chopped tomatoes and stock into the pan with the onion mixture and season. Simmer, uncovered, for a further 5 minutes.

- Stir in the cannellini beans and seafood and cook for 5–8 minutes until the fish has cooked through and is opaque. Stir in the dill.

- Spoon a little of the sauce into the pasta, then divide between two plates. Top with the remaining sauce and the rocket, and serve with the lemon and an extra drizzle of olive oil, if you like.

Mackerel parcels with a drizzle of tahini

Nothing beats this dish for simplicity – fresh mackerel keeps wonderfully fresh while baking in parchment paper so none of the protein, vitamin D or B6 is lost. Tahini cools the warming chilli (optional) and spices – and there are plenty of antioxidants in the red pepper and tomato to give the dish a glow.

DF SERVES 2   525 calories

1 tbsp olive oil	Sea salt and freshly ground black pepper
½ small red onion, finely chopped	4 small mackerel fillets
1 small tomato, finely chopped	1 tsp ground coriander
1 baby courgette, finely chopped	½ tsp ground cumin
½ small red pepper, deseeded and finely chopped	½ lemon, sliced
35g fine wholemeal bulgur wheat	2 tsp tahini, to drizzle
½ red chilli, finely chopped (optional)	Green beans, to serve (optional)

- Preheat the oven to 200°C/400°F/Gas Mark 6.

- Put the olive oil into a bowl. Add the onion, tomato, courgette, pepper, bulgur wheat and chilli, if using, and stir everything together with a tablespoon of water. Season well and stir again.

- Lay the mackerel on a board, skin side down, and rub with the coriander and cumin spices. Season with black pepper.

- Cut out two large pieces (around 35–40cm square) of non-stick baking parchment or foil and place a mackerel fillet on each. Put 2 lemon slices on each fillet and divide the bulgur wheat mixture between them. Top with the remaining fillets, to make two 'sandwiches'. Drizzle 2 tablespoons water over each pile.

- Wrap the parchment around the mackerel and secure, then transfer to a baking sheet and bake in the oven for around 20 minutes. Open the parcels and drizzle each with a teaspoon of tahini, then serve with steamed green beans.

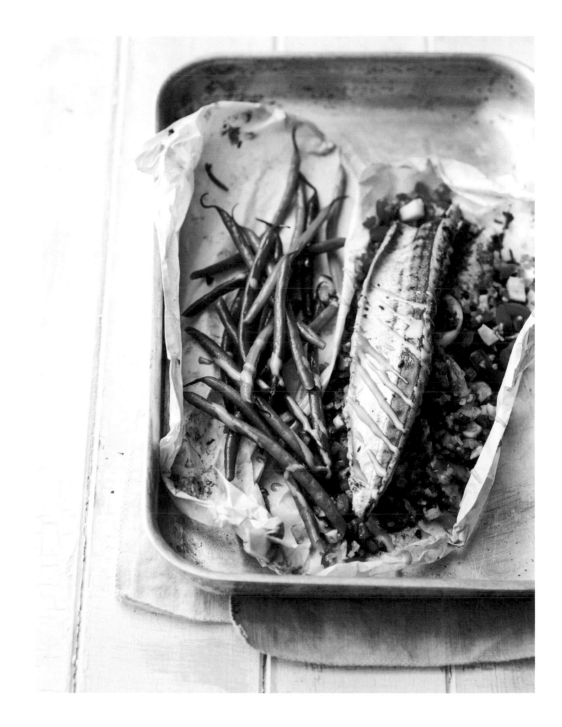

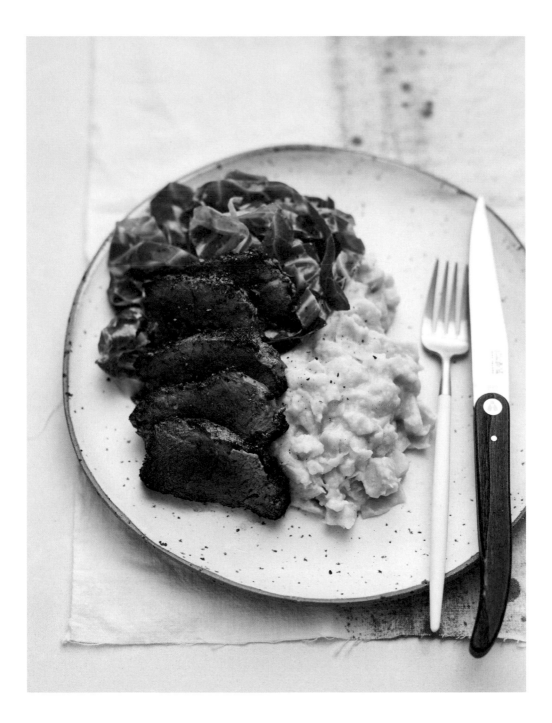

Simple steak with parsnip and butter bean mash

With my family being 100 per cent grass-fed livestock farmers (lamb and Hereford beef), high-quality meat is often on the menu in my house. Organic steak is a powerful source of iron and protein. The comforting mash of parsnip and butter beans offers soluble and insoluble fibre, while the spring greens are full of magnesium and phytoestrogens.

SERVES 2   467 calories

300g organic grass-fed fillet steak
1 tsp olive oil
½ small sprig of rosemary, leaves finely chopped
Sea salt and freshly ground black pepper
1 parsnip, unpeeled and chopped
1 shallot, chopped

200ml light vegetable or chicken stock
400g can butter beans, drained well
15g butter
1–2 tsp Dijon mustard
150g spring greens

- Put the steak into a small sealable container, drizzle over the oil then scatter with the chopped rosemary leaves. Turn the steak over so it's completely covered in the marinade. Season well, then cover and set aside.

- Put the parsnip and shallot in a medium pan with the stock. Cover and bring to the boil, then simmer for 15–20 minutes until the parsnip is very soft.

- About 5 minutes after the parsnip has started cooking, heat a frying pan until hot. Fry the steak for 2 minutes each side – top, bottom and around the outside, too – until it's done the way you like it. Take the pan off the heat, cover and set aside to allow the meat to rest.

- Add the butter beans to the parsnip halfway through cooking and continue to simmer. Once the parsnip is cooked, drain just over half the liquid from the parsnip and beans. Mash well with half the butter and the mustard.

- Bring a large pan of water to the boil and blanch the spring greens for 2–3 minutes. Drain well and add the remaining butter, then toss to coat the greens in the buttery juices.

- Divide the mash between two plates and top with the greens. Slice the steak and arrange half on each plate then drizzle over any juices from the frying pan.

Baked sweet potato burgers

I'm a big fan of the phytoestrogens provided by the kidney beans and chickpeas in these delicious veggie burgers – and they're favourites with my five children too!

(V) GF **SERVES 2**   470 calories

1 small sweet potato (around 175g), unpeeled

400g can mixed beans, drained well (or ½ x 400g can each kidney beans and chickpeas, drained well)

1 medium egg, beaten

50g gram flour or soya flour

½ tsp cayenne pepper

2 tbsp freshly chopped parsley

Sea salt and freshly ground black pepper

1 tsp olive oil

2 gherkins, halved

For the slaw:

½ small carrot, grated

½ small courgette, grated

4 cherry tomatoes, quartered

25g Cheddar cheese, grated

2 tsp olive oil

1 tsp red wine vinegar

- Preheat the oven to 200°C/400°F/Gas Mark 6.

- Chop the sweet potato – there's no need to peel – and put in a pan. Cover with cold water and put a lid on the pan. Bring to the boil and simmer for 10–15 minutes until just tender, but not too soft.

- Put the beans into a bowl with the egg, flour, cayenne and parsley. Drain the potatoes well, then leave them in a colander resting on the pan for a minute to steam. Spoon them into the bowl, season well and mash everything together.

- Heat a large frying pan until hot, then drizzle over the olive oil. Use a large spoon to divide the mixture roughly into quarters. The mixture will be quite soft, so spoon out a quarter of the mixture into a quarter of the frying pan and shape into a round. Do the same with the other portions of mixture. Cook over a medium heat for about 2 minutes until golden, then flip over and cook the other side. Transfer to a baking sheet lined with parchment and bake in the oven for 10–15 minutes until firm.

- Meanwhile, make the slaw. Mix everything together and season well. Put two burgers onto each plate and top with the gherkin. Spoon the coleslaw alongside, and serve.

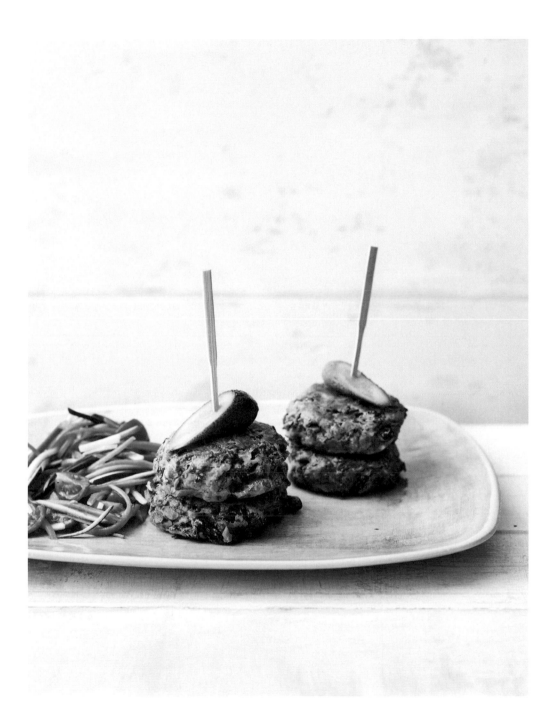

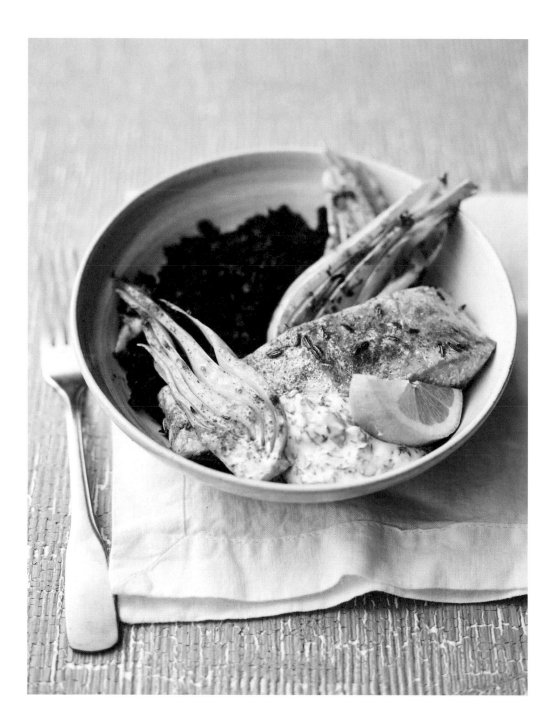

Salmon with fennel and beetroot rice

Fish and fennel are a dream match for me. I don't eat it often, but I do always buy wild or organic salmon, and oily fish is full of Omega-3 fatty acids plus vitamins B6 and B12, which both help the body use energy from food. I love this beetroot rice – it's low in carbohydrates and makes for a light alternative to regular rice. Beetroot is also a helpful liver cleanser and energy booster, while fennel aids digestion.

GF SERVES 2   463 calories

1 tbsp oil

½ tsp fennel seeds, crushed

Good pinch cayenne pepper

Sea salt and freshly ground black pepper

½ fennel bulb, cut into wedges (roughly chop the fronds, too)

2 x 150g wild or organic salmon fillets

250g beetroot, peeled

½ lemon, halved

50g plain live Greek yoghurt

1 tbsp each freshly chopped parsley, mint and basil

- Preheat the grill.

- Put the oil into a bowl and add the fennel seeds and cayenne. Season well and stir in the fronds from the fennel. Add the fennel wedges and salmon fillets and toss to coat in the oil.

- Spread the fennel and salmon out onto a baking sheet.

- Blitz the beetroot in a food processor until it looks like rice. Put in a pan and pour in 75ml water. Cover the pan with a lid and bring to a simmer. Steam for around 10 minutes, then turn off the heat. Add a squeeze of juice from one lemon quarter.

- Meanwhile, grill the fennel and salmon for around 15 minutes, turning the fennel over halfway through.

- Mix together the yoghurt and herbs and squeeze in a little more lemon juice.

- Divide the beetroot rice between two bowls, top with the salmon and fennel and yoghurt sauce, and serve with the remaining lemon quarter, cut into wedges

Spiced lamb cutlets with cauli rice pilaff

I love this dish for being both light in texture and heavy in nutrients. Besides protein, lamb is a good source of iron and zinc, while the pilaff is a clever low-carb accompaniment that uses blitzed cauliflower instead of rice to provide fibre and vitamin C. Spice it up with turmeric to add in a powerful anti-inflammatory.

GF **SERVES 2**   426 calories

4–6 organic lamb cutlets

For the marinade:
½ tsp turmeric
½ tsp ground coriander
½ tsp mild curry powder
2–3 good pinches chilli powder (optional)
1 tsp olive oil
Juice of ¼ large lemon
Sea salt and freshly ground black pepper

For the pilaff:
½ cauliflower (around 250g), roughly chopped
1 shallot, roughly chopped
2 tsp olive oil
1 tsp turmeric
1 tsp cumin seeds
3 green cardamoms, cracked slightly
1 clove garlic, sliced
100g fresh or frozen peas (thawed if frozen)

For the sauce:
50g plain live yoghurt
Sprig of mint, leaves chopped

- Mix all the ingredients for the marinade together in a shallow dish. Lay the lamb cutlets on top so that one side gets coated in the spice mix, then turn over and do the other side. Set aside to marinate.

- Put the cauliflower into a food processor with the shallot. Whizz until the cauliflower pieces have broken down into little grains that look like rice.

- Heat the oil in a pan and stir in the spices and garlic. Cook for about 1 minute, just before the garlic starts to turn golden. Spoon the cauliflower mixture into the pan and stir everything together, making sure it's coated in the spiced oil. Add the peas and 2–3 tablespoons cold water, and stir again. Reduce the heat to low and cook, covered, for 5–7 minutes until the 'rice' is tender.

- Meanwhile, heat a frying pan until hot and fry the lamb cutlets for 2–3 minutes each side until golden. Set aside to rest.

- Stir the yoghurt, mint and 2–3 teaspoons water together in a bowl. Season well.
- Once the pilaff has finished cooking, divide between two plates, top with the lamb cutlets and drizzle over the yoghurt sauce.

LIZ'S TIP

To serve this with a salad, cut 1 tomato into wedges. Put in a bowl with ¼ red onion, sliced, and a 5cm-piece of cucumber, chopped. Add a good squeeze of lemon juice, season well and toss to mix.

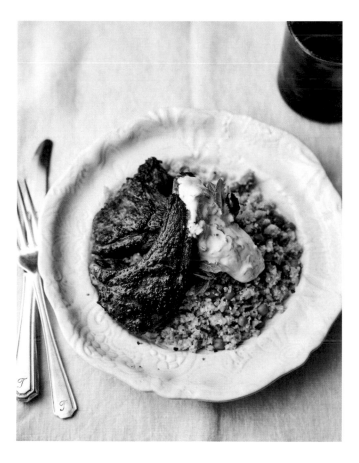

Grilled trout with spring vegetable medley

I don't think you can beat lightly baked trout, served here with vegetables also lightly cooked to keep the nutrients. The vitamin D, not to mention protein, in the trout is excellent, and there is plenty of fibre and vitamin C in the potatoes and green veggies. Asparagus wins the nutrient award with vitamin C, B6, iron and calcium, as well as being a powerful gut-friendly prebiotic.

GF **SERVES 2**   488 calories

2 tbsp olive oil, plus extra for brushing

Juice of ½ lemon

Small handful of basil leaves, plus extra to garnish

Sea salt and freshly ground black pepper

15g pecorino or Parmesan, grated

300g small new potatoes, quartered

150g asparagus tips, halved

4 stems purple sprouting or tender-stem broccoli, halved

4 spring onions, cut into 4 chunks

2 x 150g trout fillets, boned

- Preheat the grill.

- Whizz the oil, lemon juice, basil and a tablespoon of water in a small blender to make a dressing. Season with black pepper – there's no need to add any salt as the cheese can be salty – then stir in the grated cheese.

- Bring a medium pan of water to the boil and cook the potatoes for 10–15 minutes until just tender. Add the asparagus, broccoli and spring onions, cover with a lid and cook for 2–3 minutes more until the vegetables are tender.

- Brush the trout with oil and season. Transfer to a baking sheet and grill until the fish is opaque and cooked through (this should take roughly 5 minutes).

- Drain the vegetables in a colander then put them back into the pan. Add the dressing, toss everything together and divide between two plates. Top with the trout and garnish with a few extra basil leaves.

Chicken cacciatore

This hearty Italian stew has been given a menopause makeover and uses protein-boosting cannellini beans, with the lean chicken adding extra protein. Cooked tomatoes are high in lycopene, peppers are packed with beta carotene, while calcium, Omega-3 and Omega-6 are found in kale.

SERVES 2   311 calories

2 skinless chicken thighs

Sea salt and freshly ground black pepper

Cayenne pepper, to season

1 tbsp olive oil, plus a little extra for the kale

½ small onion, sliced

2 cloves garlic, sliced

½ each red and yellow pepper, deseeded and sliced

100g small chestnut mushrooms, halved

½ x 400g can chopped tomatoes

1 tbsp tomato purée

150ml chicken or vegetable stock

½ x 400g can cannellini beans, drained

6 black or green olives

2 sprigs of thyme

100g kale, chopped

Small handful of basil or parsley, chopped

- Season the chicken with salt and pepper and a good pinch of cayenne.

- Heat half the oil in a medium casserole pan and fry the chicken on each side for 2–3 minutes until golden. Lift out of the pan and set aside.

- Add the remaining oil to the pan, followed by the onion, garlic, peppers and mushrooms and continue to cook over a low to medium heat until the vegetables are starting to turn golden. Season well.

- Stir in the chopped tomatoes, tomato purée and stock, then add the beans, olives and thyme. Return the chicken to the pan, tucking it just under the sauce, and cover the pan with a lid. Bring to a simmer, then cook on a low heat for 30–40 minutes until the chicken is very tender.

- About 10 minutes before the chicken is ready, preheat the grill. Put the kale in a bowl and add a teaspoon of oil. Rub the oil into the leaves. Spread out on a baking sheet and grill until golden and starting to turn golden and crispy. You'll need to watch it like a hawk otherwise it can turn from bright green to black and burnt in what seems like an instant.

- When the stew is ready, stir in the herbs, then divide between two bowls. Scatter over the kale and serve.

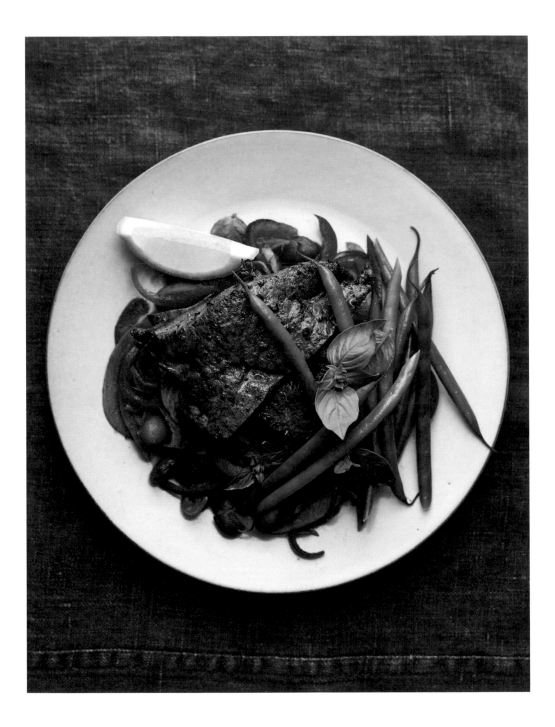

Calves' liver with peppers, onion and beans

The delicate flavours in this dish are dependent on using good organic calves' liver and cooking it gently. Liver is often overlooked but I think it's an excellent source of energy-boosting iron and vitamin B. Not only are borlotti beans full of protein and fibre, they also boast magnesium and potassium, while the peppers provide beta carotene and plenty of vitamin C. You can substitute the calves' liver for tofu, if you like.

DF GF **SERVES 2**   370 calories

4 tsp olive oil

1 small red onion, finely sliced

½ each red, yellow and orange pepper, deseeded and sliced

1 clove garlic, sliced

½ tsp cayenne pepper

1 tbsp cider vinegar

400g can borlotti beans, drained well

Small handful of fresh basil, roughly torn

Sea salt and freshly ground black pepper

1 tsp balsamic vinegar

250g calves' liver, sliced in half

150g green beans, trimmed

½ lemon, halved

- Heat a tablespoon of the oil in a medium pan and sauté the onion over a low heat for 5 minutes. Stir in the peppers. Add a tablespoon of water then continue to sauté the vegetables for 10–15 minutes, stirring every now and then.

- Stir in the garlic and cayenne and cook for 1–2 minutes, then pour in the cider vinegar and cook for a further 1–2 minutes. Add the beans and half the basil, season well and toss everything together. Simmer for a few more minutes to heat the beans through.

- Put the remaining oil into a dish and add the balsamic vinegar. Lay the liver slices in the mixture and toss to coat. Season well.

- Heat a wide frying pan over a medium heat until hot. Add the liver and pan-fry for 2–3 minutes on one side, then turn over and cook the other side.

- Bring a small pan of water to the boil and add the green beans. Simmer for 3–5 minutes until tender.

- Divide the bean sauce between two plates and top with the calves' liver, plus any juices from the pan, and the green beans. Scatter with the remaining basil and serve with a wedge of lemon to squeeze over.

Baked sweet potatoes with black beans

I can't beat this warming dish for rich colour – plus important nutrients. Sweet potatoes provide vitamin C and several B vitamins, plus are a valuable source of fibre and potassium. Black beans are full of protein, iron and magnesium, while the avocado adds good fat to boost your skin.

Ⓥ GF **SERVES 2**   400 calories

2 small sweet potatoes, unpeeled

2 tsp olive oil

½ tsp smoked paprika

Sea salt and freshly ground black pepper

½ each red and green pepper, deseeded and chopped into rough chunks

2 spring onions, chopped into rough chunks

½ x 400g can black beans, drained and rinsed

½ avocado, chopped

Small handful of parsley, chopped

50g feta cheese, crumbled

½ lime, halved

- Preheat the oven to 200°C/400°F/Gas Mark 6.

- Cut the sweet potatoes in half lengthways and score a crisscross on the cut sides of each. Mix together the oil and paprika and brush half over the sweet potatoes. Place on a baking sheet, season and bake in the oven for 15 minutes. There should be a little oil left over for the vegetables.

- After 15 minutes, spoon the peppers and spring onions into a small ovenproof dish, drizzle over the remaining spiced oil and season well. Toss the vegetables around in the oil then cook in the oven under the sweet potatoes for 30 minutes until the potatoes are golden and tender. Stir the vegetables halfway through cooking.

- Stir the black beans through the vegetables, along with the avocado and half the parsley. Put the baked potatoes onto two plates, spoon over the bean mixture, then scatter over a little feta cheese and the rest of the parsley. Serve with a wedge of lime.

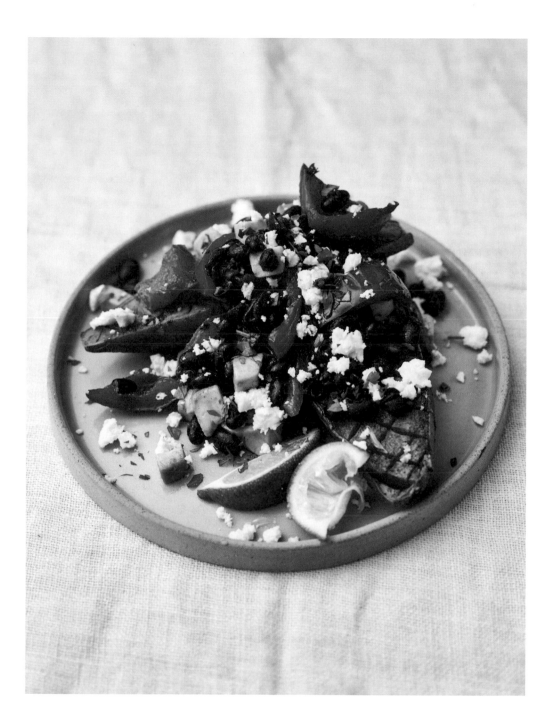

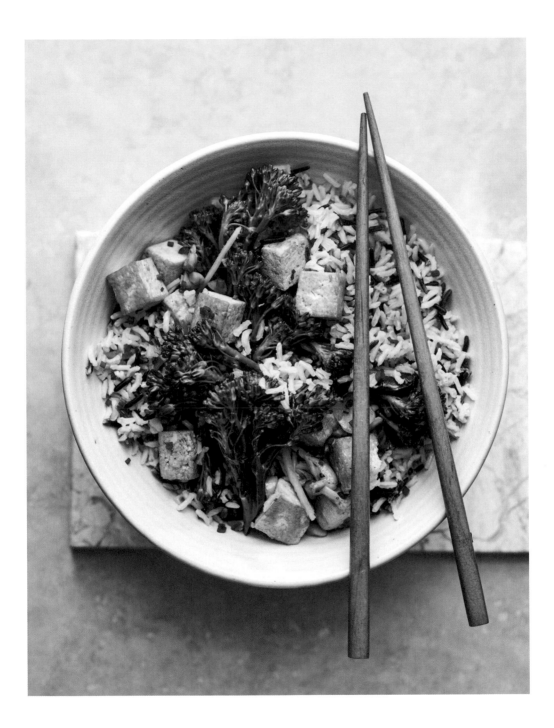

Broccoli, brown rice and tofu

For a zesty, crunchy vegetarian meal that packs in the nutrients then this works for me! Made from soya beans, tofu is a reliable vegetarian source of protein, calcium and iron, while sprouting broccoli when stir-fried retains its vitamin C and chromium content.

Ⓥ DF SERVES 2   529 calories

250g brown basmati and wild rice, rinsed well (enough for this meal and Quick-fix kedgeree, page 189)

Pinch sea salt

1 tbsp olive oil

200g tender-stem broccoli, halved

2 cloves garlic, sliced

2cm piece fresh ginger, peeled and chopped into matchsticks

1 tsp toasted sesame oil

15g cashew nuts, chopped

250g firm tofu, chopped into 2cm chunks

1 tbsp soy sauce

Small handful of chives, finely chopped

- Put the rice into a pan and cover with plenty of cold water. Add a pinch of salt, cover with a lid and bring to the boil. Simmer for 20–25 minutes until tender, and drain well.

- About halfway through the rice's cooking time, heat the olive oil in a wok or frying pan and stir-fry the broccoli for 3–4 minutes until starting to become tender. Stir in the garlic, ginger, sesame oil and cashew nuts and cook for 1 minute.

- Add 2 tablespoons water to the pan, cover with a lid and cook for 3–4 minutes until the broccoli is cooked all the way through. Add the tofu, pour over the soy sauce and scatter over the chives. Toss for a minute or two more to heat the tofu through.

- Divide half the brown rice between two bowls – set aside the other half (see tip below). Spoon the stir-fry on top and serve.

LIZ'S TIP

This recipe makes enough rice for two dishes – the other is the Quick-fix kedgeree on page 189. Spread the rice out on a plate to cool quickly (warm rice breeds bad bugs) then pack in an airtight container and chill for up to 2 days.

Herby turkey meatballs with tomato sauce and vegetable noodles

I love making meatballs and this recipe is ideal for a light supper thanks to the turkey which, as well as being low in saturated fat, high in protein and packed with B vitamins, contains tryptophan, an amino acid which aids sleep. Alongside the nutrient-dense veggies are red lentils – an excellent source of fibre, protein and boron for bone health, while L-lysine, an essential amino acid, helps with calcium absorption.

SERVES 2   380 calories

For the sauce:
1 tbsp olive oil
1 shallot, finely chopped
1 small carrot, finely chopped
1 small stalk celery, finely chopped
1 clove garlic
½ x 400g can chopped tomatoes
25g dried red lentils
300ml hot stock

For the meatballs:
250g turkey steak, chopped
Small handful of freshly chopped herbs, such as parsley, basil, thyme and rosemary, plus a few extra basil leaves to serve
Sea salt and freshly ground black pepper
25g sourdough breadcrumbs
10g Parmesan, grated

For the vegetable noodles:
1 courgette (around 175–200g)
¼–½ butternut squash (around 175–200g)

- First make the meatballs. Put the turkey into a food processor and add the herbs. Season well and whizz until the meat and herbs are finely chopped. Add the breadcrumbs and Parmesan and whizz again to mix quickly.

- Roll the mixture into 8 balls and set aside.

- Heat the oil in a medium pan and sauté the shallot, carrot, celery and garlic for 5 minutes. Stir in the tomatoes, lentils and stock, then season well and simmer, covered, for 15 minutes until the lentils are tender.

- Spoon the meatballs into the sauce and simmer for 3–5 minutes. Turn over and simmer for a further 3–5 minutes.

- Meanwhile, use a serrated Y peeler or spiraliser to create noodles out of the courgette and squash.

- Bring a medium pan of water to the boil and add a pinch of salt. As soon as it is boiling, add the noodles. Cook for 2–3 minutes then drain well.

- Divide the noodles between two plates and spoon the meatballs on top, followed by the sauce. Scatter over a few basil leaves to serve.

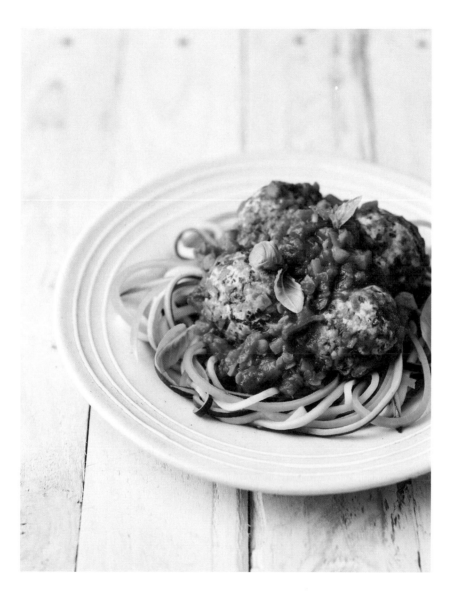

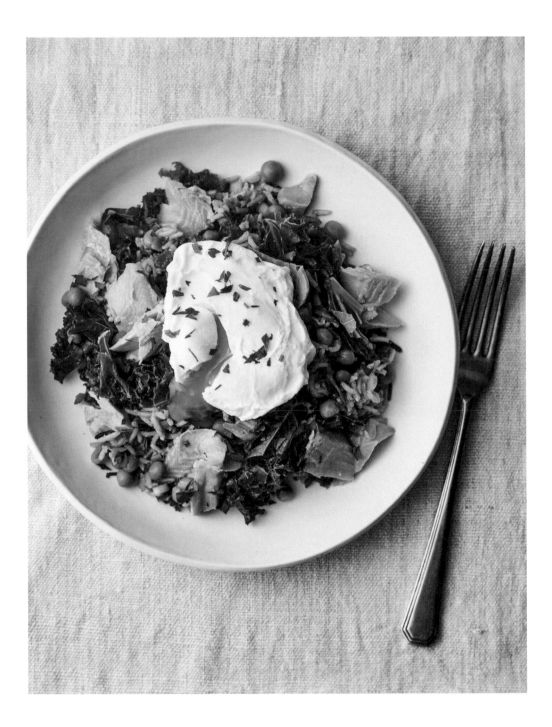

Quick-fix kedgeree

For a light nutritious meal which is also incredibly filling then look no further than my version of kedgeree, which includes kale to supply vitamin C. In addition to the texture, I use brown rice for its chromium and wild rice for its magnesium. As an oily fish, trout offers Omega-3 and vitamin D, while the eggs contain protein, biotin and chromium. One essential ingredient is turmeric, to give the dish its glow and bolster gut health.

GF SERVES 2   400 calories

150g frozen peas, thawed | Sea salt and freshly ground black pepper
100g kale, chopped | Leftover cooked brown basmati and wild rice (see
15g butter | Broccoli, Brown Rice and Tofu, page 184)
2 spring onions, chopped | 2 medium eggs
1 tsp turmeric | Small handful of chopped parsley
1 tsp mild or medium curry powder | 125g hot smoked trout fillets, flaked

- Put the peas and kale into a large bowl. Pour over enough boiling water from the kettle to cover the vegetables. Leave for 2 minutes then drain well.

- Half-fill a medium pan with water, cover with a lid and bring just to the boil.

- Melt the butter in another pan and add the spring onions, turmeric, curry powder and a tablespoon of water. Season well and stir-fry for around 3 minutes until the spring onions are just golden.

- Stir in the rice, the drained peas and kale and mix everything together. Pour over 2 tablespoons water, stir again then cover with a lid and keep over a low heat to steam and heat through.

- Once the water is boiling, turn the heat down low. Crack an egg into a small glass and carefully tip it into the just bubbling water. Do the same with the other egg. Allow to cook for 2–3 minutes until the white is set and yolk is still runny. Carefully lift out with a slotted spoon and drain well.

- Use a fork to fluff up the rice, then stir in the parsley and flaked trout. Divide between two plates, spoon the eggs on top and serve.

Green goodness broccoli and nut balls

I do like a good meatball but wanted to create a tasty meno-friendly veggie alternative, so here is a protein-packed dish. Soya flour and nuts are rich in protein, while broccoli is high in vitamin C so will boost both skin and collagen.

GF **SERVES 2** 470 calories

For the broccoli balls:
200g broccoli, roughly chopped
25g soya flour
15g whole almonds
15g brazil nuts
1 tsp flax seeds
1 red chilli, chopped
1 tsp turmeric
2–3 tbsp roughly chopped parsley
15g Parmesan, freshly grated
2–3 tbsp beaten egg

For the sides:
1 tbsp olive oil
2 small sweet potatoes, sliced into thick fingers
Sea salt and freshly ground black pepper
1 tsp red wine vinegar
½ avocado, chopped
100g tomatoes, quartered
2 tbsp freshly chopped parsley
6 olives

- Preheat the oven to 200°C/400°F/Gas Mark 6. Line a baking sheet with baking parchment. Bring a large pan of water to the boil and add the broccoli. Cook for 2–3 minutes until the broccoli is just tender. Drain well.

- Whizz the soya flour, nuts, flax seeds, chilli, turmeric and parsley in a food processor, then add the broccoli, cheese and egg. Continue to whizz until it comes together.

- Use a teaspoon to scoop up heaped portions of the mixture. Roughly shape into a round with another teaspoon then nudge onto the baking parchment. Do the same with the rest of the mixture until you've made 10–12 balls and space them apart on the baking sheet.

- Put 2 teaspoons of the olive oil into a roasting tin and add the sweet potatoes. Toss together and season well before putting in the oven along with the broccoli balls. Bake for 20–25 minutes.

- Meanwhile, put the remaining oil into a bowl with the vinegar and season well. Add the avocado, tomatoes, parsley and olives. Stir together and set aside.

- When the chips are done and the balls are cooked through, divide between two plates. Spoon the avocado salsa on the side and serve.

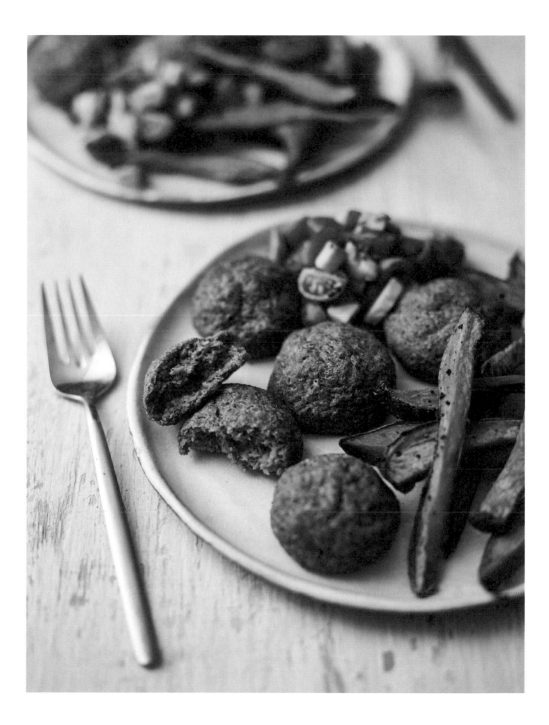

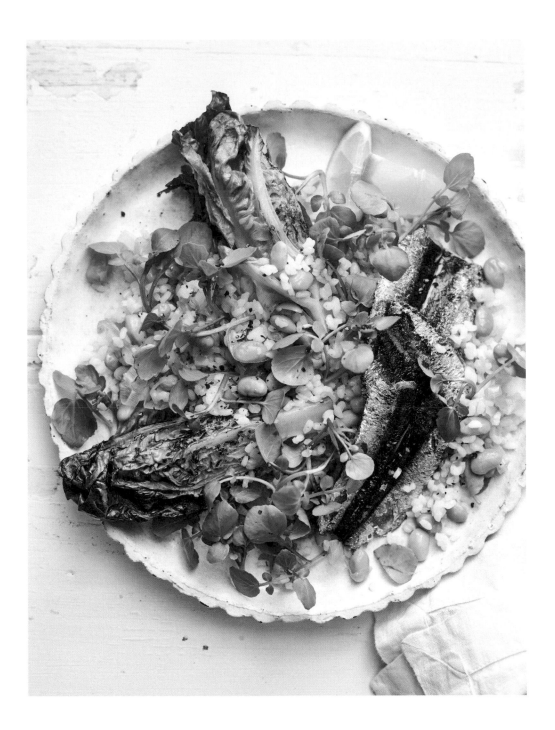

Grilled sardines with fresh summer salad

As a rich source of Omega-3, sardines are perfect – and if they are small enough I like to eat the bones too for added calcium! I prefer short-grain brown rice as an alternative carb to potatoes as it is low GI and tastes so good. Do try it if you're not familiar (I buy mine in bulk online). Add watercress and soya beans so the dish has a dash of iron and magnesium.

GF SERVES 2   400 calories

80g short-grain brown rice
4–6 sardines, cleaned and butterflied
2 tsp olive oil, plus extra for brushing
Sea salt and freshly ground black pepper
1 small, young leek, sliced
100g frozen soya beans, thawed

1 Little Gem lettuce, halved and each half cut into 3–4 wedges
10g butter
1 lemon, halved
25g watercress, chopped, plus a few sprigs to garnish

- Put the rice into a pan and add 225ml boiling water. Cover with a lid and bring to a simmer. Turn the heat down to the lowest setting and steam for 20–25 minutes until tender.

- Brush the sardines with olive oil (around a teaspoon) and season well. Preheat the grill.

- About 10 minutes before the rice is ready, heat the oil in a pan and sauté the leek for 5 minutes until golden. Add the beans and lettuce and cook for a minute or two. Add the butter to the pan and season well. Continue to cook until the lettuce has softened and is starting to turn golden.

- Put the sardines on a baking sheet and grill until golden.

- Fluff up the rice with a fork and stir into the vegetables. Squeeze in the juice from one lemon half and fold in the watercress. Taste to check the seasoning.

- Cut the other lemon half in two. Spoon the rice salad between two plates, top with the grilled sardines and serve with a few extra sprigs of watercress and a wedge of lemon.

Easy roast chicken

It's easy to associate roast chicken with roast potatoes, but here I've substituted low GI root vegetables, including beetroot to add iron, while lentils offer much-needed fibre and the amino acid L-lysine. Plenty of herbs add delicious flavour to this high-protein, low-fat lunch.

SERVES 2   560 calories

2 tbsp olive oil

Sprig each of rosemary and thyme, leaves
   chopped

Sea salt and freshly ground black pepper

150g baby turnips, halved if large

125g small beetroots, halved (or quartered if
   large)

125g Chantenay carrots

2 x 150g organic chicken breasts, skin on

75g dried puy lentils

Small handful of soft herbs, such as chives, parsley
   and basil

For the gravy:

1 tsp olive oil

10g butter

½ red onion, finely sliced

1 tsp soya flour

200ml light chicken stock

½ tsp Dijon mustard (optional)

- Preheat the oven to 200°C/400°F/Gas Mark 6.

- Pour the oil into a small bowl, add the chopped herbs and a tablespoon of water and season. Add the vegetables and turn them over in the herbs and oil until they're coated, then spoon into a small ovenproof dish or roasting tin. Add the chicken to the bowl and toss in the remaining herby oil.

- Put the vegetables in the oven and roast for 20–30 minutes. Meanwhile, heat a frying pan until hot. Add the chicken, skin side down, and pan-fry for 2–3 minutes until golden. Turn over and cook on the other side for 1 minute. Place on top of the vegetables and roast in the oven for 15–20 minutes until cooked through. The time varies, depending on how thick the chicken fillets are – to check they are done, pierce the middle of one with a sharp knife to make sure there are no pink juices or pink bits left. Keep the frying pan to make the gravy.

- Meanwhile, put the lentils in a pan and add enough cold water to cover by about a couple of centimetres. Put a lid on the pan and bring to a simmer. Cook for 20–25 minutes until tender. Set aside.

- To make the gravy, heat the oil and butter in the frying pan you used for the chicken and sauté the onion for 5 minutes until golden. Stir in the soya flour and cook for 1 minute. Stir in the stock and bring to a simmer. Simmer for 5 minutes until thickened. Whisk in the mustard, if using.

- Drain the lentils then return to the pan and stir in the soft herbs and 1–2 tablespoons of the gravy. Divide between two plates, then top with the vegetables and chicken. Spoon over the remaining gravy and serve.

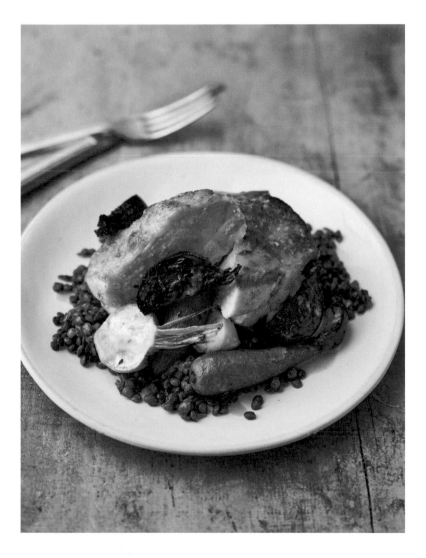

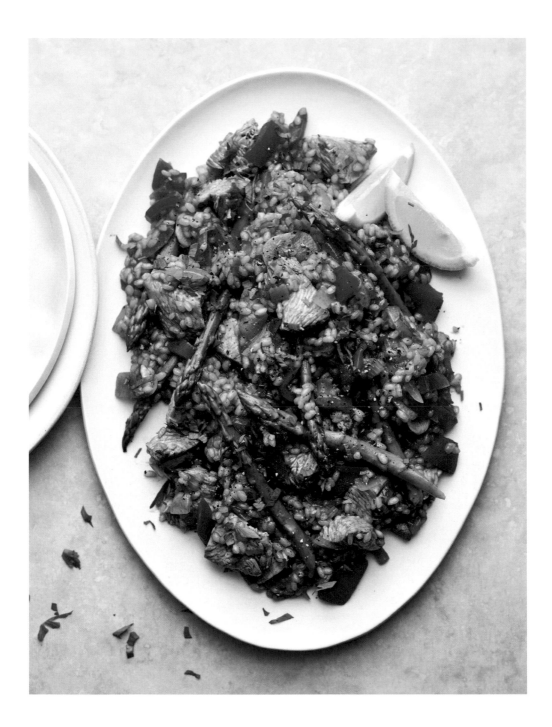

Smoky rice with turkey, red pepper and asparagus

This dish is strong on flavour and nutrients – another ideal dinner dish as turkey is full of tryptophan, the amino acid that aids sleep, while brown rice is low GI and a source of biotin.

DF SERVES 2   529 calories

1 tbsp olive oil

½ lemon, halved

1 tsp smoked paprika

Sprig of thyme, leaves only

250g turkey, roughly chopped

Sea salt and freshly ground black pepper

1 small red onion, roughly chopped

½ red pepper, deseeded and roughly chopped into chunks

1 clove garlic, sliced

150g short-grain brown rice

500ml hot light chicken stock

1 tsp tomato purée

100g asparagus (or tender-stem broccoli), halved

Small handful of freshly chopped parsley

- Put a teaspoon of the oil into a shallow dish. Squeeze in half the lemon then add half the paprika, thyme sprig and the turkey. Season and toss everything together to coat.

- Heat the remaining oil in a sauté pan and cook the onion, pepper and garlic over a low to medium heat for around 8 minutes, by which time the vegetables should be starting to turn golden.

- Stir in the rest of the paprika and cook for 1–2 minutes. Stir in the turkey and rice and cook for a further 1–2 minutes.

- Mix the stock and tomato purée together, then pour into the pan. Stir the mixture to settle the ingredients in an even layer then cover the pan with a lid and cook for 30 minutes or until the rice is tender. After 20 minutes, scatter the asparagus (or broccoli) over the top and continue to cook for the remaining time.

- Check the rice is cooked, then stir in half the parsley. Spoon the rice onto a sharing dish, scatter with the remaining parsley and serve with a squeeze of the remaining lemon.

Asian-style beef broth

I love this strong beef broth with an Asian flavour thanks to the tangy bite given by arame, a seaweed from the kelp family, which adds iodine and so boosts the metabolism. Bone-building beef is a concentrated source of protein as well as offering vitamins B6 and B12.

DF SERVES 2   202 calories

2 short ribs of organic, grass-fed beef   1 red chilli, finely sliced
10g arame dried seaweed   1 bok choy, roughly chopped
2 tbsp miso paste   ½ red pepper, deseeded and sliced
½ tsp ground white pepper   2 spring onions, finely sliced

- Preheat the oven to 170°C/325°F/Gas Mark 3.

- Put the beef short ribs into a medium ovenproof casserole pan, pour in 1 litre cold water and cover with a lid. Put the pan on the hob over a medium heat and bring to the boil. As soon as the water is boiling, transfer to the oven and cook for 3 hours until the beef is tender.

- While the beef is cooking, put the seaweed into a bowl, cover with cold water and soak for 10 minutes. Drain well.

- Lift the ribs out of the stock and cool a little before shredding the meat. Put the meat back into the stock, and stir in the miso paste and white pepper.

- Add the chilli, bok choy, pepper, spring onions and drained seaweed and place the pan over a medium heat. Simmer for 3–5 minutes until the vegetables are just tender.

- Divide between two bowls and serve.

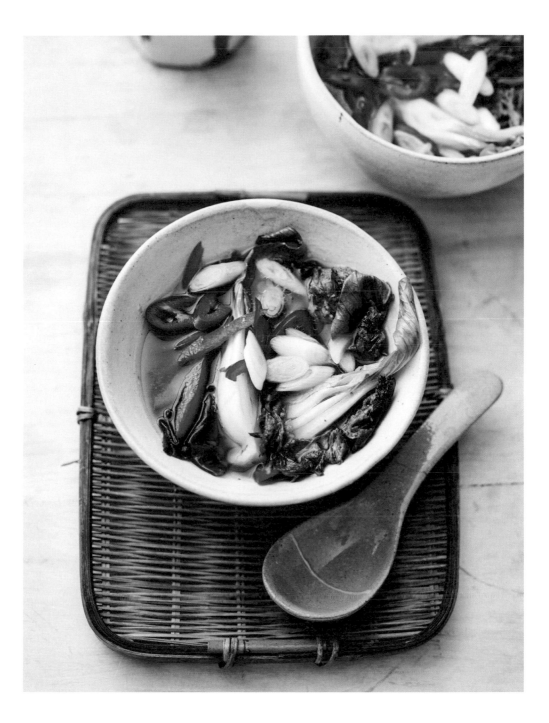

DESSERTS AND TREATS

Baked pears with walnut crumble

My family love this alternative to a traditional crumble for its soft, sweet flavours – and for me it has the added bonus of ingredients with health benefits. Pears contain boron – a mineral important for bone health, which helps to prevent osteoporosis and blood clots – and ginger boosts the immune system and circulation; while the topping includes walnuts, a great source of vitamin D, and oats for added soluble fibre.

(V) SERVES 2   296 calories

2 pears, halved or quartered and cored
Juice of ½ orange
1 tbsp honey, xylitol or stevia
1cm piece fresh ginger, peeled and cut into
  matchsticks
Plain live yoghurt, to serve

For the walnut crumble:
20g chilled butter
20g spelt flour
10g oats
15g chopped walnuts
½ tsp ground cinnamon
20g honey

- Preheat the oven to 200°C/400°F/Gas Mark 6.

- First make the walnut crumble. Rub the butter and flour together in a bowl. Fold in the oats, walnuts and cinnamon until everything is mixed evenly. Stir in the honey.

- Line a baking sheet with baking parchment and scatter over the crumble mix.

- Put the pears into an ovenproof dish. Mix the orange juice, honey (xylitol or stevia) and ginger together and pour over the top. Bake in the oven for 20–30 minutes until tender.

- Put the crumble mixture in the oven, on the shelf under the pears, and bake for 10–12 minutes until golden. Set aside to cool.

- Spoon the pears onto two plates with some of the juices – you can leave the ginger behind if you like (it's just to flavour the juice). Roughly break up the crumble and scatter over the top. Serve with a spoonful of plain live yoghurt.

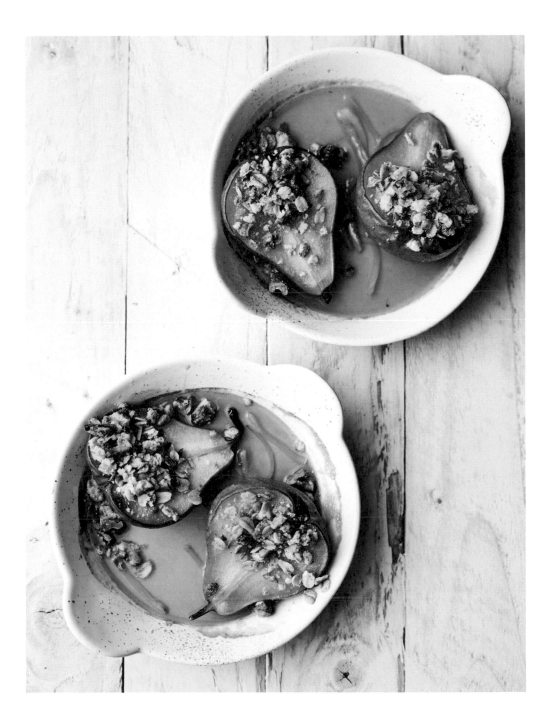

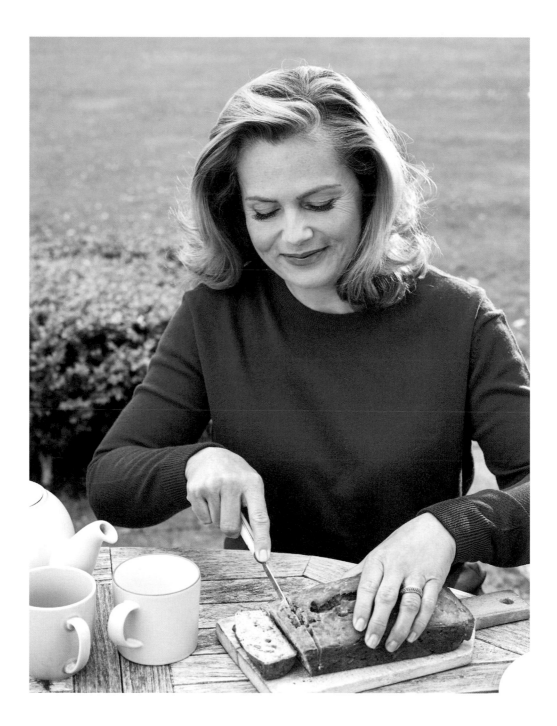

Seeded loaf

This densely packed bread is filled with nuts and seeds so that one slice is all I need. This is my go-to loaf. Spelt and soya flour are excellent alternatives to wheat when it comes to digestion – many find spelt easier to digest and soya flour is high in magnesium.

V DF CUTS INTO 8–10 SLICES   210–167 calories

For the quick starter:
½ tsp dried yeast
½ tsp honey
1 tbsp spelt flour
50ml lukewarm water

For the bread:
300g spelt flour
50g soya flour
30g mixed seeds and chopped nuts, such as flax
    seeds, sunflower seeds and flaked almonds or
    chopped walnuts
½ tsp sea salt
1 tbsp olive oil

- At least 2 hours and up to 8 hours ahead, make the quick starter. Put the ingredients into a clean jam jar. Stir everything together, then cover with a lid and set aside so that the yeast activates.

- When you're ready to bake the loaf, preheat the oven to 210°C/410°F/Gas Mark 6 ½. Lightly oil a loaf tin measuring 17 x 8cm (base) x 6cm (depth) and line with baking parchment.

- Sift the flours into a large bowl and add the seeds and nuts and sea salt. Stir together. Make a well in the middle and pour in the starter. Add the oil and 250–275ml lukewarm water and mix everything together. The dough will be looser than regular dough, more like a thick batter.

- Spoon into the prepared tin and transfer to the oven. Bake for 50–60 minutes. To check the loaf is ready, carefully take it out of the tin and tap the base – if it sounds hollow, it's done. Put on a wire rack to cool before slicing.

LIZ'S TIP

Store this loaf wrapped tightly in cling film for up to 3 days. To freeze, wrap tightly in cling film and freeze for up to 1 month. Take out of the freezer the night before you want to enjoy it so it has time to thaw.

Not-too-sweet muffins

The sweet, subtle flavours in these gorgeous muffins make a delicious alternative to sickly, soggy commercial varieties. There's no added sugar and plenty of nutrients – from fibre in the spelt flour to iron in the dried apricots, while pumpkin seeds are a good source of zinc.

(V) MAKES 6   216 calories

1 apple or pear, grated
50g Cheddar cheese, grated
1 tbsp pumpkin seeds
1 tsp sunflower seeds
2 dried apricots, finely chopped
125g spelt flour

1 tsp baking powder
2 tbsp olive oil
125g plain live yoghurt
1 medium egg
1 tbsp honey, xylitol or stevia (optional)

- Preheat the oven to 200°C/400°F/Gas Mark 6. Line a muffin tin with 6 paper cases.

- Put the apple or pear, cheese, seeds, apricots, flour and baking powder into a bowl and mix everything together. Make sure there are no clumps of the grated ingredients – you can use a fork to loosen those bits if you need to. Make a well in the middle.

- In a separate bowl, whisk together the oil, yoghurt, egg and honey (xylitol or stevia), if using, until smooth.

- Scrape all the wet mixture into the middle of the dry mixture and very quickly and deftly mix all the ingredients together until just combined. Don't overwork the mixture or the muffins will be heavy, so it's fine if you can still see a few floury patches in there.

- Spoon the mixture among the paper cases and bake for 20–25 minutes until risen and golden. Check to see if they're done by inserting a skewer into the centre of one. If it comes out clean, they're ready. Lift onto a wire rack and leave to cool.

LIZ'S TIP

Once cool, freeze leftover muffins by wrapping tightly in cling film and freezing for up to 1 month. Take out of the freezer to thaw the night before you're going to eat them.

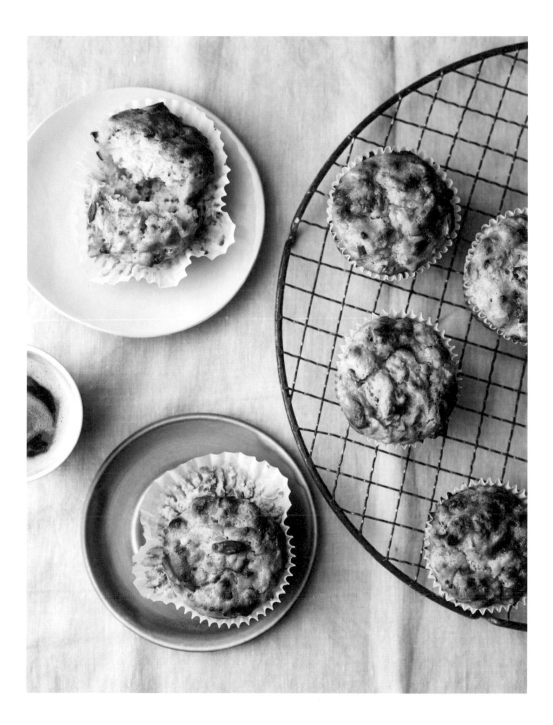

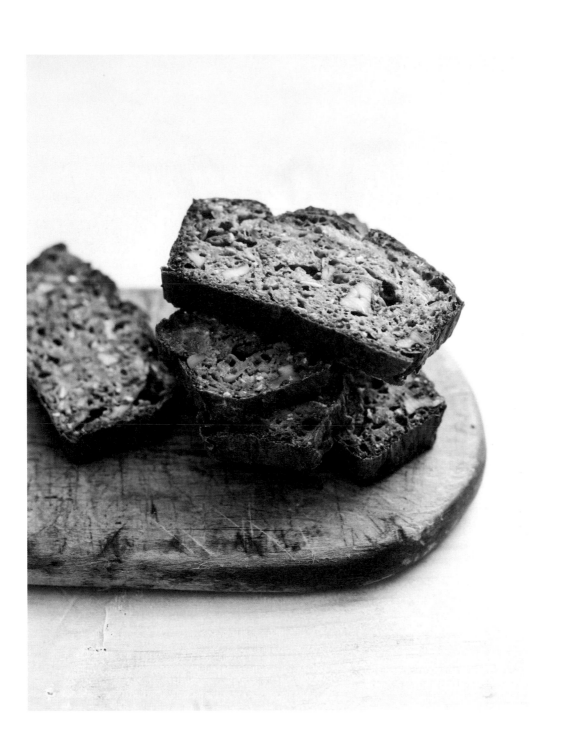

Meno-tea loaf

One bite of this rich loaf tells you that it is incredibly wholesome and packed with fruit and nuts. Where to start on the nutrients? All the dried fruits provide fibre, plus apricots contain iron and dates supply boron, while the walnuts offer calcium and vitamin D. Then there are the flax seeds (linseeds), which are fabulous for the skin and overall digestion, as well as being rich in phytoestrogens.

V DF CUTS INTO 8–10 SLICES   117–93 calories

4 dried dates, chopped

4 dried figs, chopped

4 dried apricots, chopped

6 brazil nuts, chopped

6 walnuts, chopped

2 tbsp flax seeds

150ml just-brewed Earl Grey tea

1 carrot (around 100g), grated

1 tbsp unsweetened desiccated coconut

1 tsp ground cinnamon

150g spelt flour

1 tsp baking powder

1 medium egg, beaten

125ml soya milk

- The night before you're going to make this, or up to 8 hours ahead, put the dates, figs, apricots, nuts and flax seeds into a bowl. Pour over the tea, cover and leave to soak. By the time you come to make the loaf, all the tea will have soaked into the fruit.

- When you're ready to make the loaf, preheat the oven to 200°C/400°F/Gas Mark 6. Line a 450g loaf tin with baking parchment.

- Add the carrot, coconut, cinnamon, flour, baking powder, egg and soya milk to the bowl of soaked dried fruit, nut and seed mixture and mix well. Spoon into the prepared loaf tin, and bake in the oven for 45 minutes.

- Reduce the heat to 180°C/350°F/Gas Mark 4 and bake for a further 30–45 minutes or until a skewer inserted into the centre comes out clean.

- Carefully lift out of the tin and put on a wire rack. Allow to cool before slicing.

Chocolate coconut pots

Who can resist this heavenly dessert? It's a real treat for my girlfriends, who love its intense, rich flavour – but with relatively healthy ingredients. Just take care if you're one of the unfortunate few to have dark chocolate trigger headaches – and eat at lunchtime to avoid its caffeine content interfering with sleep.

Ⓥ DF SERVES 2   381 calories

35g plain chocolate (85% cocoa), chopped

6 tbsp coconut cream

1 tsp coconut oil

1 tbsp honey or date syrup

1 medium organic egg, separated

15g toasted unsweetened coconut flakes

- Put the chocolate into a bowl with 4 tablespoons of the coconut cream, the coconut oil and half the honey or date syrup. Set the bowl over a pan of just simmering water, making sure the base doesn't touch the water, and heat until the chocolate melts. You can also do this in the microwave on the lowest heat setting.

- Add the egg yolk to the mixture, and stir in slowly.

- Whisk the egg white in a separate bowl until thick and mousse-like. Fold into the chocolate mixture.

- Divide between two small glasses and chill for 2 hours until set.

- Serve topped with the remaining coconut cream and sprinkled with the toasted coconut flakes.

LIZ'S TIP

You can also serve this with a few cacao nibs sprinkled over the top.

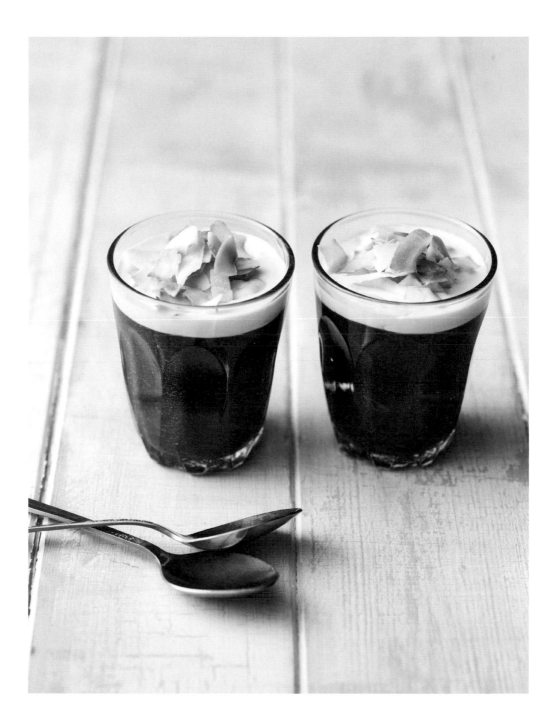

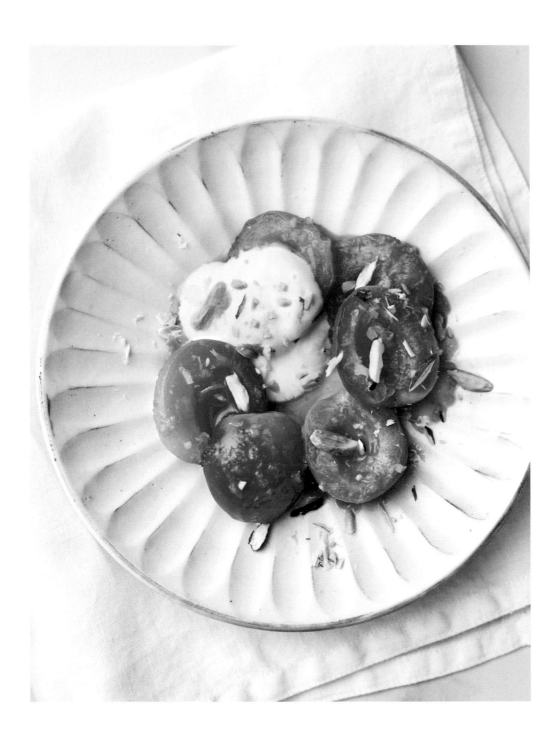

Simple poached apricots

This pretty dessert ticks all the boxes for being both sweet and nutritious. Fresh apricots are packed with iron, fibre and vitamin C. They are also one of the lowest fruits for fructose (the natural fruit sugar). I add in warming fresh ginger to dishes whenever I can – it gives the immune system a real boost and is an anti-inflammatory like its root cousin, turmeric.

(V) GF **SERVES 2**   215 calories

2 tbsp honey	6 apricots, halved and stoned
Zest and juice of 1 orange	2 tbsp plain live Greek yoghurt
4cm piece fresh ginger, peeled and chopped	8 whole almonds, roughly chopped and toasted

- Put the honey, orange zest and juice and ginger into a small pan. Add the apricots and pour in 200ml water. Bring to the boil, then simmer for 5 minutes.

- Remove the apricots and set aside, then turn the heat to medium and cook the juices until they reduce to a syrup. This will take around 4–5 minutes.

- Divide the apricots between two bowls, drizzle with the syrup, top with the yoghurt and almonds and serve.

LIZ'S TIP

For an extra-powerful probiotic boost, stir 1–2 tablespoons plain kefir into the yoghurt (see page 218).

Summer berry slump

This gorgeous summer pudding has been given a healthy twist with spelt flour, for iron and magnesium, and wheatgerm for added fibre. It has no added refined sugar and only healthy fats in the shape of olive oil, while the berries are knockout for both vitamin C and antioxidants.

V **DF** SERVES 2   507 calories

For the fruit base:
250g frozen berries
1 tbsp raw, mild-flavoured honey
1 tsp ground cinnamon
1 tsp cornflour

For the sponge 'slump':
50ml olive oil
1 medium egg
35g raw, mild-flavoured honey
1 tsp vanilla extract
50g spelt flour
1 tbsp wheatgerm
½ tsp baking powder
15g hazelnuts, finely chopped
Plain live Greek yoghurt, to serve

- Preheat the oven to 200°C/400°F/Gas Mark 6.

- Put the berries into a pan and add 50ml water, the honey and cinnamon. Cook over a medium heat until the juices start to run. Put the cornflour into a small bowl, add a tablespoon of water and stir until smooth. Pour into the pan and stir into the fruit mixture. Simmer for 1–2 minutes until the juices thicken slightly. Spoon into a small ovenproof dish and set aside.

- Put the olive oil, egg, honey and vanilla extract into a bowl and whisk together until smooth. Fold in the flour, wheatgerm, baking powder and half the hazelnuts.

- Spoon the sponge mixture onto the berries. It'll be soft like a batter but don't worry, it's meant to be like that. Scatter over the remaining hazelnuts and put the dish onto a baking sheet. Transfer the baking sheet and dish to the oven and bake for 18–20 minutes until the sponge is a rich golden colour on top. Serve with a spoonful of Greek yoghurt.

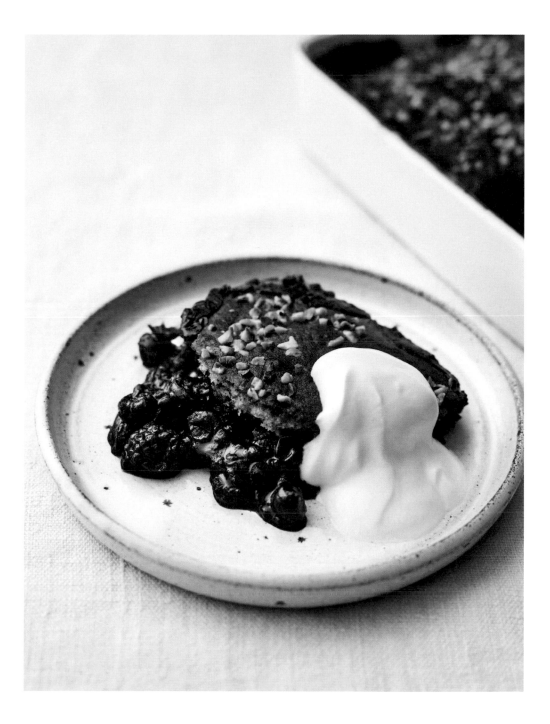

DRINKS

Kefir

I am a huge fan of probiotic supplements and there are easy ways to boost your own good-gut bacteria – one is by making kefir. The fermented yoghurt taste is an acquired one (especially if you keep it for too long as the flavour strengthens), but trust me on this one – you will feel fantastic for drinking it. Not only does it dramatically enhance beneficial gut bacteria, it also helps heal inflammatory ailments, including eczema and rosacea, which can worsen during times of hormonal change. The most effective kind is made with dairy milk (cow, goat or sheep), but you can use coconut milk (from a carton, not a can) or oat milk.

V GF **MAKES AROUND 1 LITRE**   126 calories per 200ml serving

5g sachet kefir starter culture, such as Nourish Kefir	1 litre high-quality milk (I use organic, pasture-fed whole milk)

- Start by mixing a little of the milk with the powder to dissolve. Stir for 10 minutes to combine all the cultures with the milk. Then pour in the rest of the milk and stir again for a further 10 minutes. Yes – you really do need to stir for this long to combine all the cultures and prevent the mixture from separating into lumps as it ferments. I find the gentle stirring process calmingly therapeutic and do this while listening to music or my favourite Wellbeing podcast.

- Cover with a cloth and leave at room temperature for about 12 hours (I leave mine overnight). When ready, the kefir will have thickened slightly. Give it a good stir and pour into a lidded container to keep in the fridge. It keeps for up to a week – but the flavour will intensify. Not to be missed!

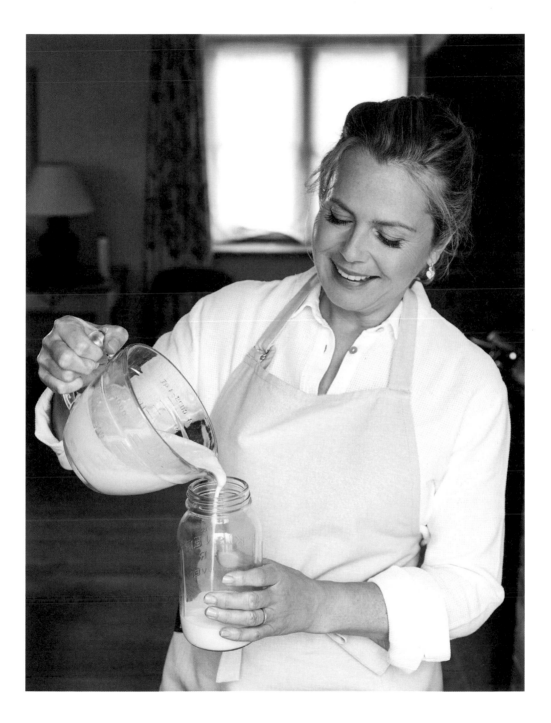

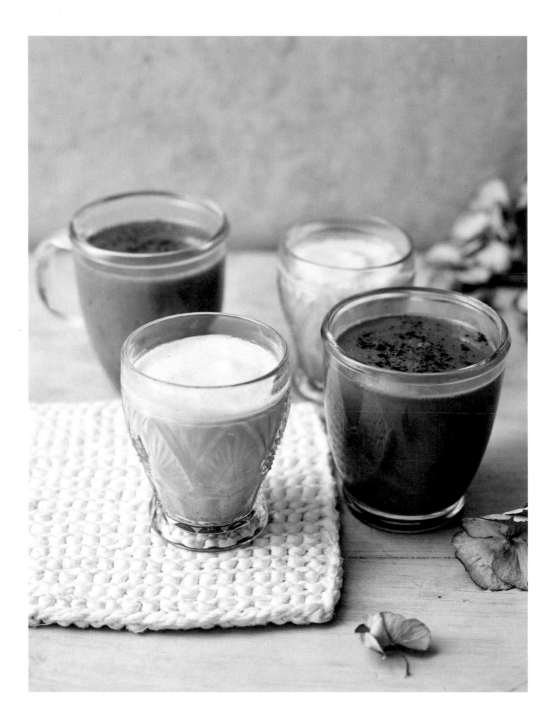

Spiced hot chocolate

I love this spiced hot chocolate which has no added sugar — just plenty of dark chocolate which is full of antioxidants, iron and magnesium. Laced with cinnamon to help pep up the metabolism, it also boosts beneficial gut bacteria. Just don't drink in the evening as the high caffeine content of the dark chocolate may further disturb sleep (and obviously avoid if sensitive to dark chocolate).

V GF SERVES 2   200 calories

300ml dairy or oat milk (make your own by simply soaking porridge oats in cold water)

2 tsp coconut oil

30g plain chocolate (85% cocoa), grated

4 cardamom pods, crushed

½ tsp ground cinnamon, plus a little extra to serve

- Pour the milk into a pan and bring to the boil. Add the coconut oil, chocolate, cardamom pods and cinnamon and stir everything together.

- With the heat on a medium setting and the milk just simmering, stir well for 3–4 minutes until the chocolate has melted.

- Divide between two heatproof glasses and sprinkle over a little extra cinnamon to serve.

Turmeric chai latte

The aromatic and warming flavours of this drink give me such a lift whatever time of day I make it. The spices each have their own health-giving properties – turmeric is a brilliant anti-inflammatory, ground ginger is a source of iron and magnesium, and cinnamon can help curb sugar cravings, thus hopefully removing the temptation to eat a biscuit at the same time! See page 220 for photograph.

(V) GF **SERVES 1**   96 calories

2–8 cardamom pods, seeds only
¼–½ tsp turmeric
½ tsp ground cinnamon

½ tsp ground ginger
150–200ml dairy, oat, nut or soya milk

- Crush the cardamom seeds in a pestle and mortar until finely ground. Scrape into a glass. Add the turmeric, cinnamon, ginger and 2 tablespoons boiling water and stir together.

- Heat the milk in a pan until just boiling. Whisk well until frothy. Pour onto the turmeric spice mixture and stir again to mix everything together.

Sage tea

You can of course buy sage tea in the supermarket but homemade tastes completely different and I think so much more delicious. Why is sage known for soothing hot flushes? It can lower inflammation throughout the body, boost the immune system and may even help prevent the onset of diabetes. It's also a comforting pick-me-up.

V DF GF SERVES 1   5 calories

4 sage leaves
2 slices fresh ginger
1 slice lemon, halved

- Put the sage, ginger and lemon into a small tea pot or jug. Pour hot water over the top and leave to steep for 5 minutes.

- Strain into a mug and serve.

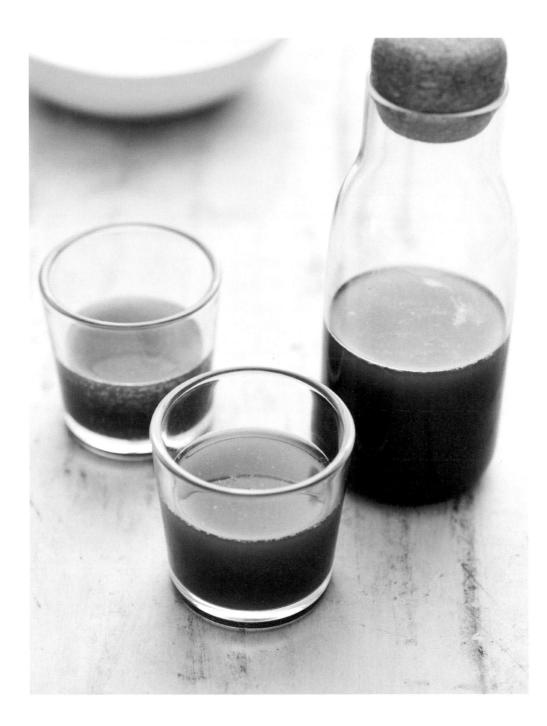

Homemade lemon and ginger kvass

Kvass is an increasingly popular fermented drink that tastes a little like flat, slightly sour lemonade. If that doesn't sound too appealing, try it for its gut-health enhancing properties above all. It really does grow on you and I find it a useful alternative to sugar-laden fizzy drinks packed with phosphates that leach calcium from already vulnerable bones. You can make kvass with all kinds of flavourings: lemon and ginger is a good combo, as is apple and ginger or rhubarb and mint during the summer months.

V DF GF **MAKES AROUND 1 LITRE**   424 calories per recipe

1.2 litres lukewarm water

50g molasses sugar

100g raw organic honey

20g raisins

½ tsp dried yeast

100g fresh ginger, chopped

1 lemon, chopped

- Pour the water into a sealable plastic container and add the rest of the ingredients. Stir well to dissolve the molasses sugar and honey.

- Cover with the lid and leave on the side in the kitchen at room temperature, stirring every now and then to 'burp' the fizzing, fermenting liquid. After a couple of days, take a large metal spoon and scoop off the foam, raisins, ginger and lemon on top and add to the compost heap (if you have one).

- Strain into sterilised bottles and chill overnight. Store in the fridge and drink within a week.

Super skin-saving smoothie

If I'm going to make a smoothie I love to add extras which make it even more worthwhile to drink. Besides the vitamin C and antioxidants in these low GI fruits, I throw in spoonfuls of collagen and hyaluronic acid, as when consumed on a regular basis they can also help give skin, joints and bones a boost.

GF SERVES 1   96 calories

50g raspberries

50g blueberries

50g strawberries

1 scoop collagen powder (or according to packet instructions)

1 tsp hyaluronic acid (or according to packet instructions)

50g plain live yoghurt

- Put the berries into a mini food processor or blender. Add the collagen, hyaluronic acid and yoghurt and whizz until smooth.

- Add 200ml water and whizz again to blend all the ingredients together.

- Pour into a glass and serve.

> **LIZ'S TIP**
>
> Make this the night before to have an instant, energising breakfast in the morning. Just pour into a sealable container and chill. Don't leave it in the fridge for too long, though, or the ingredients will start to separate. Stir well before drinking.

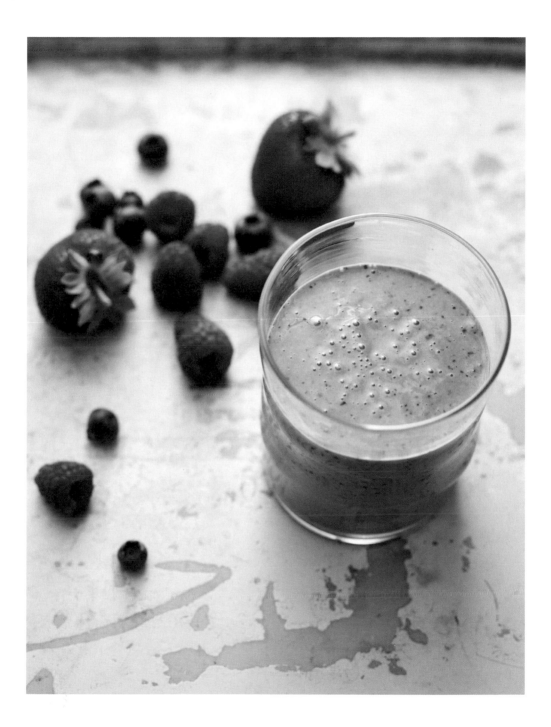

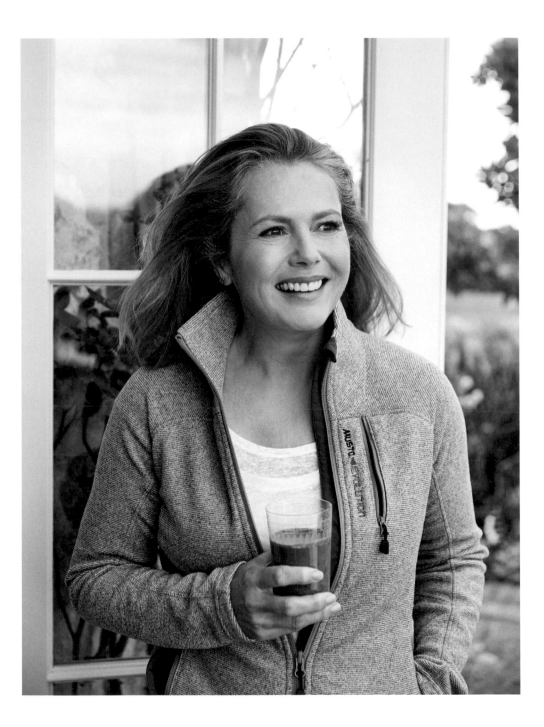

Chocolate protein shake

I love the creamy chocolate flavour of this shake which makes a special post-gym body reviver or occasional mid-morning pick-me-up, with its combination of cocoa, which is known for its iron, magnesium and calcium, and sweet blueberries, a low GI fruit high in vitamin C and brimming with antioxidants. The protein powder and plain live yoghurt both ramp up the protein content to bolster muscle mass (which in turn helps speed the metabolism), while the almond butter and coconut oil are a delicious way of using good fats in a drink.

V GF **SERVES 2**   349 calories

2 tbsp organic cocoa powder
3 tbsp almond butter
100g blueberries
150g plain live yoghurt

2 tbsp non-whey protein powder
1 tsp coconut oil
1 tsp vanilla extract
4–6 ice cubes (if you like your shake chilled)

- Put the cocoa powder into the bowl of a mini food processor or blender, then add the almond butter, blueberries, yoghurt, protein powder, coconut oil and vanilla extract.

- Whizz to blend everything together. Add 200ml water and whizz again until smooth.

- Divide between two glasses and serve with ice, if you like.

LIZ'S TIP

You can also use almond milk for a richer flavour. To make your own, put 50g whole almonds in a bowl and pour over 75ml water. Leave to soak for at least 4 hours and up to 8 hours. Drain well. Put in a food processor with 200ml cold water and whizz until the nuts have been finely ground and the water looks milky. Strain through a sieve into a bowl, pushing the mixture down with the back of a spoon to extract all the liquid. Measure in a jug and top up with extra water if you need to. Keep in the fridge and always use within 48 hours.

References

CHAPTER ONE: PERIMENOPAUSE 40+

1. Office of National Statistics 2016.
2. *New Scientist*, 25 January 2017/Journal reference: Human Reproduction, DOI: 10.1093/humrep/dew350
3. 2001: Perimenopause, depressive disorders, and hormonal variability. Center for Women's Mental Health, Perinatal and Reproductive Psychiatry Clinical Research Program, Massachusetts General Hospital, Harvard Medical School, USA. Am J Clin Nutr June 2017 105: 1493-1501; First published online May 10, 2017. doi:10.3945/ajcn.116.145607
4. University College London study. http://dx.doi.org/10.1136/bjsports-2013-092993
5. Hederstierna C, et al. The menopause triggers hearing decline in healthy women. Hear. Res. (2009), DOI: 10.1016/ j.hcares.2009.09.009
6. *Obstetrics & Gynecology*. November 1996; 88(5):785-91. The effects of smoking on ovarian function and fertility during assisted reproduction cycles. Van Voorhis BJ, Dawson JD, Stovall DW, Sparks AE, Syrop CH, Department of Obstetrics and Gynecology, University of Iowa College of Medicine, Iowa City, USA; Massachusetts General Hospital/New study tightens the link between smoking and early menopause/ScienceDaily, 16 July 2001/www.sciencedaily.com/releases/2001/07/010716112326.htm>
7. First published 10 May 2017, DOI: 10.3945/ajcn.116.14560
8. *Neurology*, October 2010.
9. Menopause/North American Menopause Society/31 May 2017

CHAPTER TWO: SYMPTOMS

1. The European Menopause Survey 2005: Women's perceptions on the menopause and postmenopausal hormone therapy. *Gynecological Endocrinology*, July 2006; 22(7): 369–375.
2. Massimiliano de Zambotti, Adrian R. Willoughby, Stephanie A. Sassoon, Ian M. Colrain, and Fiona C. Baker. Menstrual Cycle-Related Variation in Physiological Sleep in Women in the Early Menopausal Transition. *Journal of Clinical Endocrinology & Metabolism*, June 2015 DOI: 10.1210/jc.2015-1844
3. Sedentary lifestyle in middle-aged women is associated with severe menopausal symptoms and obesity. *Menopause*, 2016; 1 DOI: 10.1097/GME.0000000000000575
4. www.ncbi.nlm.nih.gov/pmc/articles/PMC4110168

CHAPTER THREE: HRT

1. Wickelgren I. Estrogen stakes claim to cognition. *Science*, 1997; 276:675–678. PubMed Citation; Tang MX, Jacobs D, Stern Y, et al. Effect of estrogen during menopause on risk and age at onset of Alzheimer's disease. *Lancet*, 1996; 348:429–432. PubMed Abstract; Paganini-Hill A, Henderson VW. Estrogen replacement therapy and risk of Alzheimer's disease. *Archives of Internal Medicine*, 1996; 156:2213–2217. PubMed Abstract; Henderson VW, Watt L, Buckwater JG, et al. Cognitive skills associated with estrogen replacement in women with Alzheimer's disease. *Psychoneuroendocrinology*, 1996; 21:421–430. PubMed Abstract.

CHAPTER FOUR: BONE HEALTH

1. HRT and oral discomfort, https://doi.org/10.1016/0378-5122(91)90279-Y
2. A review of studies published in the *American Journal of Clinical Studies*. Robert P Heaney and Donald K Langman, 2008.
3. Eamon J Laird, Trinity College Dublin.

CHAPTER SIX: SEX (AND RELATIONSHIPS)

1. Menopause/Wake Forest Baptist Medical Center, Winston-Salem, North Carolina.
2. Source: Avis NE, Colvin A, Karlamangla AS, et al. Change in sexual functioning over the menopausal transition. *Menopause*, 2016.
3. 2009 national survey of 5,045 older adults published in *Journal of Sexual Medicine*, 2010;7[suppl 5]:315–329.
4. Kuh D, et al. Urinary incontinence in middle-aged women; childhood enuresis and other lifetime risk factors in British prospective cohort. *Journal of Epidemiology and Community Health*, 1999; 53:453–458.

CHAPTER SEVEN: EMOTIONS

1. Depression and emotional aspects of the menopause. Issue: BCMJ, Vol. 43, No. 8, October 2001, 463–466. Articles Diana Carter, MBBS18. Schneider LS, Small GW, Hamilton SH, et al. Estrogen replacement and response to fluoxetine in a multicenter geriatric depression trial. Fluoxetine collaborative study group. *American Journal of Geriatric Psychiatry* 1997; 5:97– 106. PubMed Abstract.
2. European Menopause and Andropause Society's journal *Maturitas*, King's College London psychologists Beverley Ayers PhD and Myra Hunter PhD, and Staffordshire University psychologist Mark Forshaw PhD.
3. Women over 50: Psychological Perspectives, *Springer, 2007*.
4. Faculty of Occupational Medicine/Guidance on menopause and the workplace http://www.fom.ac.uk/health-at-work-2/information-for-employers/dealing-with-health-problems in the workplace/advice-on-the-menopause
5. *American Journal of Nutrition* 2015.
6. *Alternative Therapies in Health and Medicine*, November–December 2012; 18(6):11–8. Massage increases oxytocin and reduces adrenocorticotropin hormone in humans. Morhenn VI, Beavin LE, Zak PJ; *Journal of Physical Therapy Science*, October 2016; 28(10):2703–2707. Epub 28 October 2016.
7. The effect of a scalp massage on stress hormone, blood pressure, and heart rate of healthy female. Kim IH: Effects of scalp massages on stress hormones, blood pressure, and heart rate of middle-aged women with office jobs. Korean J Sports Sci, 2013, 22: 1173–1182.

Resources

Lizearlewellbeing.com – Liz's own website to bookmark for updates and ongoing features on the latest on all aspects of a healthy lifestyle and sign up to a free weekly newsletter.

RESOURCES

The British Menopause Society, thebms.org.uk
The Menopause Exchange, menopause-exchange.co.uk
Menopausesupport.co.uk
The Daisy Network, daisynetwork.org.uk (for POI)
Early Menopause Support Network, earlymenopause.com
Red Hot Mamas – In Charge of Change, redhotmamas.org
International Osteoporosis Foundation, iofbonehealth.org
British Association of Aesthetic Plastic Surgeons (BAAPS), baaps.org.uk
Relate, relate.org.uk

HEALTH PROFESSIONAL CREDITS

Dr Louise Newson, menopausedoctor.co.uk
Cognitive behavioural therapist (CBT) Anna Albright, annaalbright.com
GP and sexual dysfunction expert, Dr Anand Patel, sexmedicine.co.uk
Sleep specialist, Dr Michael Breus, thesleepdoctor.com
Physiologist and sleep therapist, Dr Nerina Ramlakhan, drnerina.com
Cosmetic surgeon Olivier Amar, olivieramar.co.uk
Neuropsychiatrist, Dr Louann Brizendine, thefemalebrain.com
Gynaecologist Dr Sara Gottfried, saragottfriedmd.com
Gynaecologist Dr Rebecca Booth, veneffect.com
Personal trainer Michael Garry, michaelgarry.london
Body Control Pilates founder, Lynne Robinson, bodycontrolpilates.com
Yoga teacher Barbara Currie, barbaracurrie.com
Celebrity dentist, Dr Richard Marques, wimpolestreetdental.com
Osteopath Nick Cowan, nickcowanosteopath.co.uk

FURTHER READING

The Venus Week by Rebecca Booth MD (Telemachus Press, 2014)
The Hot Topic by Christa D'Souza (Short Books, 2016)
The Hormone Connection by Gale Maleskey and Mary Kittel (Rodale Books, 2001)

With special thanks to Olivia Morris, Emma Marsden and Sarah Hartley. Also to Kerry September, Jonothon Malone and Lily Earle for their invaluable make-up, hair and styling.

CONVERSION CHARTS

OVEN TEMPERATURE GUIDE

	Elec ºC	Elec ºF	Elec ºC (Fan)	Gas mark
Very cool	110	225	90	¼
	120	250	100	½
Cool	140	275	120	1
	150	300	130	2
Moderate	160	325	140	3
	170	350	160	4
Moderately hot	190	375	170	5
	200	400	180	6
Hot	220	425	200	7
	230	450	210	8
Very hot	240	475	220	9

LIQUID MEASUREMENTS (under 1 litre)

Metric	Imperial	Australian/US
25ml	1 fl oz	
60ml	2 fl oz	¼ cup
75ml	3 fl oz	
100ml	3½ fl oz	
120ml	4 fl oz	½ cup
150ml	5 fl oz	
180ml	6 fl oz	¾ cup
200ml	7 fl oz	
250ml	9 fl oz	1 cup
300ml	10½ fl oz	1¼ cups
350ml	12½ fl oz	1½ cups
400ml	14 fl oz	1¾ cups
450ml	16 fl oz	2 cups
600ml	1 pint	2½ cups
750ml	1¼ pints	3 cups
900ml	1½ pints	3½ cups

WEIGHT MEASUREMENTS

Metric	Imperial
10g	½ oz
20g	¾ oz
25g	1 oz
40g	1½ oz
50g	2 oz
60g	2½ oz
75g	3 oz
110g	4 oz
125g	4½ oz
150g	5 oz
175g	6 oz
200g	7 oz
225g	8 oz
250g	9 oz
275g	10 oz
350g	12 oz
450g	1 lb
700g	1½ lb
900g	2lb

LIQUID MEASUREMENTS (over 1 litre)

Metric	Imperial	Australian/US
1 litre	1¾ pints	1 quart or 4 cups
1.2 litres	2 pints	
1.4 litres	2½ pints	
1.5 litres	2¾ pints	
1.7 litres	3 pints	
2 litres	3½ pints	

General Index

Recipe Index

About Liz

Liz Earle MBE is one of Britain's most respected and trusted authorities on wellbeing. The award-winning author of over 30 best-selling books on nutrition, diet, beauty and natural healthcare, she co-founded the eponymous global beauty brand Liz Earle Beauty Co. in 1995, before moving back to writing and broadcasting, now publishing the leading quarterly magazine *Liz Earle Wellbeing*.

An expert in feel-good food and eating well to look good, her straightforward, balanced and well-researched approach has earned her a place as a trusted visionary in the world of wellbeing. With a passion for demystifying science and sharing wellness wisdom, Liz's measured voice of reason has a deservedly large and loyal following in print, on digital, on TV and online.

Travelling the globe for research, Liz comes home to roost on an organic farm in the UK's West Country with her husband and five children.

Sign up to Liz's free *Wellbeing* newsletter with new gut- and menopause-friendly recipes and advice: www.lizearlewellbeing.com

Also by Liz Earle

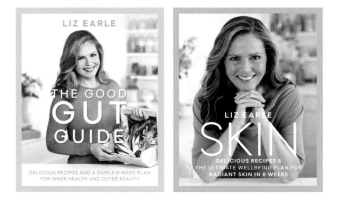

FOLLOW LIZ

 Facebook: Liz Earle Wellbeing

 Pinterest: Liz Earle Wellbeing

 Instagram: @LizEarleWellbeing

Twitter: @LizEarleWb

 YouTube: Liz Earle Wellbeing

Podcast: Wellness with Liz Earle